GLORIOUSTINA ESSIA

Herbal Encyclopedia

The Complete A–Z Profiles and Uses of Medicinal and Culinary Herbs

This book was professionally typeset on Reedsy.
Find out more at reedsy.com

Contents

GRATITUDE

My Dear Reader,

I want to extend the warmest thanks to you, my dear reader. Your choice to read my book is not just a support for my work—it's a testament to our shared belief in the power of nature and its promise of healing. Your role in this shared belief is invaluable and deeply appreciated.

This book is more than just pages bound together—it's a conversation, a shared walk through the garden of natural wisdom that has long been the backdrop of my life. Our mutual exploration of the lush possibilities of green healing fills me with an indescribable gratitude.

I've poured my dedication into these pages, hoping they'd resonate with you, offer comfort, and perhaps guide you to discover the potent balm that nature offers. I sincerely hope that this book continues to be a source of inspiration and healing for you.

INTRODUCTION

Welcome to the "Herbal Encyclopedia: The Complete A–Z Profiles and Uses of Medicinal and Culinary Herbs," a definitive guide that bridges the ancient world of herbal wisdom with modern culinary and medicinal applications. In these pages, you will explore the multifaceted world of herbs, uncovering their profound abilities to heal, nourish, and enhance our lives.

At the heart of this encyclopedia is a deep reverence for the natural world and an understanding of herbs' significant role throughout human history. From the healing fields of traditional medicine to the aromatic kitchens of the culinary arts, herbs have been integral to cultures around the globe. This book aims to illuminate the full spectrum of herbal knowledge, providing readers with detailed profiles of each herb, including its botanical characteristics, historical uses, medicinal properties, and culinary applications.

We delve into the rich tapestry of herbal lore and science, exploring how these natural wonders can address modern health challenges, enhance culinary experiences, and promote overall wellness. Each herb's profile is a meticulous compilation of research, traditional knowledge, and practical uses, ensuring readers have a well-rounded understanding of its potential.

As you navigate through the alphabetized entries, from the familiar garlic and ginger to the lesser-known yet equally intriguing herbs like ashwagandha and yarrow, you will discover the unique stories and benefits each herb offers. This encyclopedia doesn't just list facts; it invites you to explore the practical aspects of incorporating these herbs into your daily routine, whether as natural remedies, culinary enhancements, or sources of personal enrichment.

"Herbal Encyclopedia" is designed for a wide audience, from healthcare professionals and herbalists to home cooks and gardeners. It serves as a practical reference, a source of inspiration, and a gateway to the natural world's healing and culinary possibilities.

HERBS A: PROFILES AND USES

Acacia (Acacia spp.)

- **Profile:** Acacia, also known as gum Arabic, is a thorny tree native to Africa and parts of Australia.
- **Uses:** The sap is a dietary fiber and a soothing agent in traditional medicine. It's also used in pharmaceuticals, food, and textile industries as a stabilizer and emulsifier.

Acerola (Malpighia emarginata)

- **Profile:** Also known as Barbados Cherry, Acerola is a tropical fruit-bearing shrub.
- **Uses:** The fruit is extremely rich in vitamin C and is used to prevent vitamin C deficiency, improve immune function, and as an antioxidant.

Achiote (Bixa orellana)

- **Profile:** Achiote, or annatto, is a shrub or small tree originating from the tropical region of the Americas.
- **Uses:** Its seeds are a natural coloring agent in food and cosmetics. Traditional uses include treating burns and infections and as an insect repellent.

African Mango (Irvingia gabonensis)

- **Profile:** A tree native to Central and West Africa, known for its edible mango-like fruits.
- **Uses:** The seed extract is popular in weight loss supplements. It's also used for its potential benefits in managing diabetes and cholesterol.

Agar (Gelidium amansii)

- **Profile:** Agar is a gelatinous substance obtained from red algae.
- **Uses:** Commonly used as a laxative, a vegetarian gelatin substitute in cooking, and microbiology for culturing bacteria.

Agave (Agave spp.)

- **Profile:** A genus of succulent plants known for their rosette growth and spiky leaves.
- **Uses:** Agave nectar is used as a natural sweetener. The sap, known as aguamiel, is believed to have anti-inflammatory and antimicrobial properties.

Agrimony (Agrimonia eupatoria)

- **Profile:** A perennial herb found in temperate regions, known for its slender spikes of yellow flowers.
- **Uses:** Traditionally used for its astringent properties to treat mild diarrhea, as a throat gargle, and topically for skin inflammation.

Ale Hoof (Glechoma hederacea)

- **Profile:** Also known as ground ivy, this herb is a creeping member of the mint family.
- **Uses:** Traditionally used to treat respiratory conditions, such as bronchitis

and asthma, and as a tonic for the digestive system.

Alfalfa (Medicago sativa)

- **Profile:** A perennial flowering plant often used as forage for livestock.
- **Uses:** In herbal medicine, it's used for its nutrient-rich leaves and sprouts, beneficial for conditions like arthritis and kidney problems, and to increase breast milk production.

Allspice (Pimenta dioica)

- **Profile:** The dried unripe fruit of the Pimenta dioica tree, native to the Greater Antilles and Central America.
- **Uses:** Used primarily as a spice in cooking, allspice has also been used in traditional medicine for digestive issues, as a pain reliever, and for its anti-inflammatory properties.

Aloe Vera (Aloe barbadensis)

- **Profile:** A succulent plant famous for its thick, fleshy leaves.
- **Uses:** Widely known for its soothing, healing properties, particularly for burns, sunburns, and skin irritations. Also used internally for digestive health.

Althea (Althaea officinalis)

- **Profile:** Also known as the marshmallow plant, it's a perennial species indigenous to Europe, Western Asia, and North Africa.
- **Uses:** Its roots and leaves are used for their mucilaginous properties to soothe mucous membranes, treat coughs, and for skin health.

Amur Cork Tree (Phellodendron amurense)

- **Profile:** A tree native to East Asia, known for its thick corky bark.
- **Uses:** The bark is used in traditional Chinese medicine for its anti-inflammatory and antioxidant properties, often for treating pain and boosting immune function.

Andrographis (Andrographis paniculata)

- **Profile:** An herbaceous plant known as the "King of Bitters."
- **Uses:** Used for its immune-boosting and anti-inflammatory effects, particularly in treating colds, flu, and upper respiratory infections.

Angelica (Angelica archangelica)

- **Profile:** A tall, aromatic plant that has been used in traditional herbal medicine as well as in cooking.
- **Uses:** Angelica root is known for its digestive stimulating effects and has been used to treat indigestion, gas, and colic. It's also been used for respiratory ailments and as an expectorant.

Anise Seed (Pimpinella anisum)

- **Profile:** A flowering plant native to the eastern Mediterranean region and Southwest Asia.
- **Uses:** Anise seed is used to treat digestive issues, relieve menopausal symptoms, and for its licorice-like flavour in cooking and beverages.

Argan Oil (Argania spinosa)

- **Profile:** Extracted from the kernels of the argan tree, native to Morocco.
- **Uses:** Primarily used in skin and hair care products for its moisturizing and nourishing properties. It's also consumed for its potential cardiovascular

benefits.

Arnica (Arnica montana)

- **Profile:** A perennial, herbaceous plant with yellow, daisy-like flowers.
- **Uses:** Used topically in creams and ointments for bruises, sprains, and muscle aches. It is not recommended for internal use due to toxicity.

Arrowroot (Maranta arundinacea)

- **Profile:** A tropical tuber plant known for its starchy rhizomes.
- **Uses:** Arrowroot powder is used as a digestive aid, a natural thickening agent in cooking, and for its soothing effect on irritated mucous membranes.

Arsemart (Artemisia vulgaris)

- **Profile:** Commonly known as mugwort, this plant is part of the daisy family.
- **Uses:** Mugwort has been used in traditional medicine for its calming effects on the nervous and digestive systems. It's also been used in various cultures for menstrual irregularities and as a dream herb.

Artichoke (Cynara scolymus)

- **Profile:** A type of thistle cultivated as food.
- **Uses:** The leaves improve digestion and liver health and lower cholesterol levels.

Ashwagandha (Withania somnifera)

- **Profile:** An evergreen shrub commonly used in Ayurvedic medicine.
- **Uses:** Known as an adaptogen, it's used to help the body resist stressors, improve energy levels, and support overall health and well-being.

Astragalus (Astragalus membranaceus)

- **Profile:** A traditional Chinese medicinal herb known for its immune-boosting properties.
- **Uses:** Used to prevent and treat colds, enhance energy and stamina, and support cardiovascular health.

Avocado (Persea americana)

- **Profile:** A tree native to South Central Mexico, known for its creamy fruit.
- **Uses:** The fruit is highly nutritious and used for its cardiovascular benefits. Avocado oil is used for its skin moisturizing and nourishing properties.

HERBS B: PROFILES AND USES

Balloon Flower (Platycodon grandiflorus)

- **Profile:** A flowering plant known for its balloon-like buds.
- **Uses:** The root is used in traditional Korean medicine to treat coughs and colds due to its anti-inflammatory and expectorant properties.

Balmony (Chelone glabra)

- **Profile:** A herbaceous plant with white or pink flowers.
- **Uses:** Traditionally used by Native Americans for liver problems and as a laxative. It has bitter properties that stimulate digestion.

Balsam Fir (Abies balsamea)

- **Profile:** An evergreen tree whose needles and resin are used in traditional medicine.
- **Uses:** The resin, known as Canada balsam, is used topically for cuts, burns, and sores. The oil is used for respiratory conditions and as an anti-inflammatory.

Basil (Ocimum basilicum)

- **Profile:** A fragrant herb commonly used in cooking, particularly in Italian cuisine.
- **Uses:** Besides culinary uses, basil is known for its anti-inflammatory properties and is used in traditional medicine to treat digestive disorders and alleviate stress.

Barberry (Berberis vulgaris)

- **Profile:** A shrub with sharp thorns and sour-tasting berries.
- **Uses:** The bark and berries improve digestion, treat gastrointestinal infections, and support liver function. It contains berberine, known for its antimicrobial activity.

Bayberry (Myrica cerifera)

- **Profile:** A shrub native to North America, known for its aromatic leaves and berries.
- **Uses:** The root bark is used in traditional medicine as an astringent to treat diarrhea and help reduce fever. Also used as a gargle for sore throats.

Bay Leaf (Laurus nobilis)

- **Profile:** An aromatic leaf from the bay laurel tree, commonly used as a seasoning.
- **Uses:** In herbal medicine, bay leaf is used for its digestive and anti-inflammatory properties. It is also believed to have a calming effect and help with respiratory issues.

Bearberry (Arctostaphylos uva-ursi)

- **Profile:** Also known as uva ursi, this plant produces small red berries.
- **Uses:** The leaves are used primarily for urinary tract infections due to their antiseptic properties. They contain arbutin, which has antimicrobial properties.

Beechdrops (Epifagus virginiana)

- **Profile:** A parasitic plant that grows on the roots of beech trees.
- **Uses:** In traditional medicine, it has been used for digestive issues and mouth sores, though it is not widely used today.

Beetroot (Beta vulgaris)

- **Profile:** A root vegetable with a deep red colour, known for its earthy flavour and nutritional value.
- **Uses:** Beetroot boosts stamina, improves blood flow, and lowers blood pressure. It also contains antioxidants and nutrients like folate, potassium, and iron.

Bergamot (Monarda spp.)

- **Profile:** A flowering plant known as bee balm for its fragrant leaves and flowers.
- **Uses:** The leaves and flowers make calming tea and treat digestive issues. Bergamot oil from the citrus fruit of the same name is used in aromatherapy.

Beth Root (Trillium erectum)

- **Profile:** Also known as red trillium or wake-robin, it is a plant with a deep red flower.
- **Uses:** Traditionally used for menstrual disorders, to relieve childbirth pains, and as a general tonic for the female reproductive system.

Bilberry (Vaccinium myrtillus)

- **Profile:** A small berry closely related to the blueberry and rich in antioxidants.
- **Uses:** Used for improving vision, including night vision. It is also used for circulatory problems and has anti-inflammatory and blood sugar-stabilizing effects.

Birch (Betula spp.)

- **Profile:** A tree known for its distinctive white bark and leaves that turn yellow in autumn.
- **Uses:** Birch leaves are used for their diuretic and anti-inflammatory properties. Birch sap is consumed as a tonic and for its minerals and vitamins.

Bistort (Polygonum bistorta)

- **Profile:** An herbaceous plant with a twisted root and spikes of pink flowers.
- **Uses:** It is traditionally used as an astringent to tighten tissues and stop bleeding. Also used for digestive disorders.

Biting Stonecrop (Sedum acre)

- **Profile:** A low-growing plant with succulent leaves.
- **Uses:** It is historically used for its anti-inflammatory and diuretic properties, but it should be used cautiously due to its irritant effects when ingested.

Bitter Apple (Citrullus colocynthis)

- **Profile:** A plant producing a small, round fruit resembling a watermelon but is extremely bitter.
- **Uses:** Used in traditional medicine as a powerful laxative and purgative. Due to its potent effects, it should be used with caution.

Bitter Orange (Citrus aurantium)

- **Profile:** A citrus tree that produces bitter oranges for their rind and oil.
- **Uses:** Bitter orange extract is used in weight loss supplements and as an appetite suppressant. The oil is used in aromatherapy for anxiety and sleep disorders.

Bitter Root (Lewisia rediviva)

- **Profile:** A small plant with a pink or white flower and a bitter root.
- **Uses:** Traditionally used by Native Americans to stimulate appetite and treat gastrointestinal issues.

Bitter Sweet (Solanum dulcamara)

- **Profile:** A vine in the nightshade family with purple flowers and red berries.
- **Uses:** Used in small doses in traditional medicine to treat skin diseases such as rheumatism and as a diuretic. Due to its toxicity, it's not commonly

used today.

Blackberry (Rubus spp.)

- **Profile:** A widely known fruit-bearing bush.
- **Uses:** The berries are rich in vitamins, minerals, and fibre. The leaves and roots have been used as a traditional remedy for diarrhoea, sore throats, and wounds.

Blackberry Lily (Belamcanda chinensis)

- **Profile:** A plant with orange flowers and blackberry-like seed clusters.
- **Uses:** The rhizomes are used in traditional Chinese medicine for their anti-inflammatory and expectorant properties.

Black-Eyed Susan (Rudbeckia hirta)

- **Profile:** A North American coneflower with bright yellow petals and a dark brown centre.
- **Uses:** Traditionally used for its immune-stimulating and anti-inflammatory properties.

Black Cohosh (Actaea racemosa)

- **Profile:** A flowering plant native to North America, known for its tall white flowers.
- **Uses:** Commonly used to treat menopausal symptoms such as hot flashes, mood disturbances, and sleep disturbances.

Black Haw (Viburnum prunifolium)

- **Profile:** A shrub or small tree with clusters of white flowers and black fruits.
- **Uses:** The bark is used for its antispasmodic properties, particularly to prevent miscarriage and to treat menstrual cramps and spasmodic dysmenorrhea.

Black Horehound (Ballota nigra)

- **Profile:** A perennial herb with an unpleasant odour.
- **Uses:** It is used for its soothing and antiemetic properties to treat nausea, vomiting, and nervous system disorders.

Black Root (Veronicastrum virginicum)

- **Profile:** Also known as Culver's root, named for its dark-coloured rhizomes.
- **Uses:** Used traditionally as a laxative and to treat liver disorders.

Black Walnut (Juglans nigra)

- **Profile:** A tree known for its valuable wood and edible nuts.
- **Uses:** The hulls of the black walnut are used to treat parasitic worm infections. Also used topically for fungal infections.

Bladderwrack (Fucus vesiculosus)

- **Profile:** A type of seaweed found on the coasts of the North Sea, the western Baltic Sea, and the Atlantic and Pacific Oceans.
- **Uses:** Rich in iodine, it is often used to support thyroid health. Also used for weight loss, arthritis, joint pain, and digestive issues.

Blessed Thistle (Cnicus benedictus)

- **Profile:** A thistle-like plant with yellow, thorny flowers.
- **Uses:** Used traditionally as a digestive tonic and for treating liver and gallbladder diseases.

Bletilla (Bletilla striata)

- **Profile:** An orchid with striking purple flowers.
- **Uses:** The tubers are used in traditional Chinese medicine to stop bleeding and to heal wounds.

Bloodroot (Sanguinaria canadensis)

- **Profile:** A plant with a distinctive reddish sap.
- **Uses:** Traditionally used as an expectorant and to treat respiratory problems. It's also been used in toothpaste and mouthwash for its plaque-inhibiting properties.

Blue Cohosh (Caulophyllum thalictroides)

- **Profile:** A flowering plant native to North America.
- **Uses:** Used traditionally to ease childbirth due to its antispasmodic properties. Also used for menstrual cramps and to regulate the menstrual cycle.

Blue Flag (Iris versicolor)

- **Profile:** A perennial plant with beautiful blue flowers.
- **Uses:** Historically used for its laxative effects and to treat skin conditions. It also detoxifies the body, particularly the liver and lymph system.

Blue Vervain (Verbena hastata)

- **Profile:** A tall plant with spikes of small purple flowers.
- **Uses:** Used for its nerve-calming effects to alleviate anxiety and stress. Also used for digestive health and as an expectorant for respiratory conditions.

Buckthorn Bark (Rhamnus cathartic)

- **Profile:** Bark from the buckthorn tree, known for its strong laxative properties.
- **Uses:** Used in small doses as a natural laxative for short-term constipation relief. It should be used cautiously due to its potency.

Burdock Root (Arctium lappa)

- **Profile:** A biennial plant with long, dark roots and large leaves.
- **Uses:** Traditionally used as a blood purifier to treat skin conditions like eczema and psoriasis. Also believed to aid digestion and act as a diuretic.

Butterbur (Petasites hybridus)

- **Profile:** A perennial shrub found in Europe and parts of Asia and North America.
- **Uses:** Used to prevent migraine headaches, treat hay fever symptoms, and treat gastrointestinal issues. It must be processed to remove potentially harmful chemicals.

Bog Myrtle (Myrica gale)

- **Profile:** A small shrub with aromatic leaves.
- **Uses:** Traditionally used as an insect repellent and for its astringent properties. Also used in brewing certain traditional beers and ales.

Bogbean (Menyanthes trifoliata)

- **Profile:** An aquatic plant with trifoliate leaves and white, fluffy flowers.
- **Uses:** Used for its bitter properties to stimulate appetite and digestion. Also used for rheumatic conditions.

Boldo (Peumus boldus)

- **Profile:** An evergreen shrub native to Chile and Peru.
- **Uses:** The leaves are used to treat digestive disorders and liver conditions due to their stimulating effect on bile production.

Boneset (Eupatorium perfoliatum)

- **Profile:** A perennial plant with white, fuzzy flowers.
- **Uses:** Traditionally used to treat fever and as an immune stimulant. Also used for its anti-inflammatory and laxative effects.

Borage (Borago officinalis)

- **Profile:** A plant with star-shaped blue flowers known for its cucumber-like flavour.
- **Uses:** Used for its anti-inflammatory properties and to treat respiratory infections. Also believed to elevate mood and adrenal function.

Boswellia (Boswellia serrata)

- **Profile:** A tree native to India known for its fragrant resin, which has many medicinal uses.
- **Uses:** The resin, known as Indian frankincense, reduces inflammation in conditions like arthritis, asthma, and inflammatory bowel diseases. It's also used in incense and traditional ceremonies.

Brooklime (Veronica beccabunga)

- **Profile:** An aquatic plant with succulent leaves and small blue flowers.
- **Uses:** It is traditionally a vitamin-rich spring tonic for its mild diuretic and expectorant properties.

Brown Mustard (Brassica juncea)

- **Profile:** A mustard plant with a pungent taste, used for its seeds.
- **Uses:** Mustard seeds are used as a spice for their warming and circulatory-stimulating effects. Mustard plasters are used to treat chest congestion.

Buchu (Agathosma betulina)

- **Profile:** A plant from South Africa with a strong, minty aroma.
- **Uses:** The leaves treat urinary tract infections and as a natural diuretic. It is also used for its anti-inflammatory properties.

Bugleweed (Lycopus virginicus)

- **Profile:** A plant with a mint-like appearance and small white or purple flowers.
- **Uses:** Traditionally used to treat hyperthyroidism, anxiety, and heart palpitations due to its mild sedative effects.

Burnet Saxifrage (Pimpinella saxifraga)

- **Profile:** A plant with finely divided leaves and white flowers.
- **Uses:** Used for its digestive and diuretic properties. Also used as a treatment for coughs due to its expectorant properties.

Butcher's Broom (Ruscus aculeatus)

- **Profile:** A small evergreen shrub with flat shoots resembling leaves.
- **Uses:** Used to improve circulation, particularly for haemorrhoids and varicose veins, due to its vasoconstrictor and anti-inflammatory properties.

HERBS C: PROFILES AND USES

Calumba (Jateorhiza palmata)

- **Profile:** A climbing plant native to East Africa, known for its thick, fleshy roots.
- **Uses:** Traditionally used as a digestive tonic to treat nausea and upset stomach. Its bitter compounds stimulate digestive juices.

Calendine (Chelidonium majus)

- **Profile:** Also known as greater celandine, it has yellow flowers.
- **Uses:** Historically used to support liver health and in treating digestive issues. It has also been used topically for warts and skin lesions.

California Poppy (Eschscholzia, California)

- **Profile:** A bright orange wildflower native to the United States and Mexico.
- **Uses:** Used as a mild sedative and sleep aid. It can help relieve anxiety and tension without the addictive properties of stronger sedatives.

Cambogia (Garcinia cambogia)

- **Profile:** A small, pumpkin-shaped fruit known for its weight loss properties.
- **Uses:** Hydroxy citric acid (HCA) extract is used in weight loss supplements. It's believed to inhibit fat production and suppress appetite.

Camphor Tree (Cinnamomum camphora)

- **Profile:** An evergreen tree producing camphor, a substance used in medicinal and aromatic products.
- **Uses:** Camphor is used topically to relieve pain, irritation, and itching. It has a cooling effect and is used in some decongestant remedies.

Capsicum (Capsicum spp.)

- **Profile:** Includes various peppers, from sweet bell peppers to hot chilies.
- **Uses:** Capsaicin, found in hot peppers, is used topically for pain relief. Edible peppers are rich in vitamins and antioxidants and are believed to have metabolic-boosting properties.

Caraway Seed (Carum carvi)

- **Profile:** A biennial plant with crescent-shaped seeds commonly used in cooking.
- **Uses:** Caraway seeds have carminative properties, aid digestion, relieve flatulence, and treat gastrointestinal disorders.

Carob (Ceratonia siliqua)

- **Profile:** A flowering evergreen tree producing edible pods.
- **Uses:** Carob is a chocolate substitute rich in fiber and antioxidants. It's used for digestive health and can help with diarrhea.

Carom Seeds (Trachyspermum ammi)

- **Profile:** Small, pungent seeds used in Indian cooking.
- **Uses:** Known for digestive benefits, they treat indigestion, flatulence, and colic. Also used in traditional cough remedies.

Cardamom (Elettaria cardamomum)

- **Profile:** A spice made from the seeds of a plant in the ginger family.
- **Uses:** Besides culinary uses, cardamom treats digestive issues and bad breath and is a diuretic. It also has antioxidant and anti-inflammatory properties.

Cascara Sagrada (Rhamnus purshiana)

- **Profile:** A species of buckthorn native to North America.
- **Uses:** Used as a natural laxative due to compounds called anthraquinones that stimulate bowel movements. It should be used with caution and not for prolonged periods.

Castor Bean (Ricinus communis)

- **Profile:** A plant known for its large, glossy leaves and seed pods.
- **Uses:** Castor oil, extracted from the seeds, is used as a laxative to induce labor. It's also applied topically for skin health and to promote hair growth. The seeds are toxic and should not be ingested.

Catmint (Nepeta cataria)

- **Profile:** Commonly known as catnip, it's a perennial herb.
- **Uses:** In humans, it's used for its mild sedative properties, aiding relaxation and sleep. It's also known for its effect on cats, inducing a temporary euphoria.

Cat's Claw (Uncaria tomentosa)

- **Profile:** A woody vine found in the tropical jungles of South and Central America.
- **Uses:** Used for its anti-inflammatory properties to treat arthritis digestive system disorders and boost the immune system.

Cayenne Pepper (Capsicum annuum)

- **Profile:** A hot chili pepper is used to flavor dishes.
- **Uses:** Medicinally, it's used to boost circulation, aid digestion, and as a pain reliever when applied topically. It's also used in detox regimens.

Celery (Apium graveolens)

- **Profile:** A marshland plant that's a common food vegetable.
- **Uses:** Used for its diuretic and anti-inflammatory properties. Also believed to help lower blood pressure and aid in digestion.

Centaury (Centaurium erythraea)

- **Profile:** A small plant with pink flowers, part of the gentian family.
- **Uses:** Traditionally used as a bitter tonic to stimulate appetite and digestion. Also used for its anti-inflammatory and antifungal properties.

Chaga (Inonotus obliquus)

- **Profile:** A fungus that grows on birch trees, resembling a dark clump of dirt.
- **Uses:** Consumed as a tea, Chaga is rich in antioxidants and is used to support immune health and for its potential anti-cancer properties.

Chamomile (Matricaria chamomilla)

- **Profile:** A flowering plant known for its soothing, apple-like fragrance.
- **Uses:** Widely used in herbal teas for relaxation and sleep aid. Also used topically for skin irritations and inflammations.

Chasteberry (Vitex agnus-castus)

- **Profile:** A small berry from the chaste tree.
- **Uses:** Used primarily for menstrual disorders, PMS symptoms, and to help balance female hormones.

Cherry (Prunus spp.)

- **Profile:** Fruit-bearing trees are known for their delicious red fruits.
- **Uses:** Cherries are rich in antioxidants and are consumed for their anti-inflammatory properties, particularly in treating gout and muscle soreness.

Chervil (Anthriscus cerefolium)

- **Profile:** A delicate annual herb related to parsley.
- **Uses:** Chervil is used in traditional folk medicine to lower blood pressure and as a mild diuretic. It's also used to aid digestion.

Chickweed (Stellaria media)

- **Profile:** A common garden weed with small, star-shaped flowers.
- **Uses:** Traditionally used topically for skin conditions like rashes and eczema and internally for its mild diuretic properties and to soothe the digestive tract.

Chicory (Cichorium intybus)

- **Profile:** A perennial herbaceous plant with bright blue flowers, known for its coffee substitute.
- **Uses:** Chicory root is high in inulin, a type of prebiotic fiber, and is used to improve digestive health. It's also used for liver and gallbladder support.

Chittem Bark (Rhamnus purshiana)

- **Profile:** Also known as Cascara Sagrada, a species of buckthorn.
- **Uses:** Used as a natural laxative to treat constipation. It stimulates bowel movements by irritating the colon.

Chives (Allium schoenoprasum)

- **Profile:** A small, bulbous herb related to onions and garlic.
- **Uses:** Primarily used as a culinary herb. It's known for its mild stimulant, diuretic, and antiseptic properties in herbal medicine.

Chlorella (Chlorella spp.)

- **Profile:** A single-celled green algae that is a superfood.
- **Uses:** Rich in proteins, vitamins, and minerals, it's a dietary supplement for detoxification, boosting the immune system, and improving cholesterol levels.

Chokecherry (Prunus virginiana)

- **Profile:** A fruit-bearing shrub or small tree native to North America.
- **Uses:** The berries are used to make syrups and jams. Medicinally, they are used for colds and coughs and as a laxative. The bark is used in traditional medicine for respiratory ailments.

Cicely (Myrrhis odorata)

- **Profile:** A tall herb with sweet-smelling foliage and white flowers.
- **Uses:** The leaves and seeds are used in cooking and traditional medicine for their expectorant properties and to sweeten bitter herbal concoctions.

Cilantro (Coriandrum sativum)

- **Profile:** An herb with a distinctive, fresh taste, known for its leaves and seeds (coriander).
- **Uses:** Used in cooking for its flavor. It's known for its digestive, anti-inflammatory, and blood sugar-regulating properties.

Cinchona Bark (Cinchona spp.)

- **Profile:** The bark of a tree native to South America is known as the source of quinine.
- **Uses:** Quinine extracted from cinchona bark is used to treat malaria. It's also used for its digestive and analgesic properties.

Cinnamon (Cinnamomum spp.)

- **Profile:** A spice obtained from the inner bark of several tree species.
- **Uses:** Used for its flavor in cooking and baking. It's recognized for its antioxidant, anti-inflammatory, and blood sugar-lowering effects.

Cleavers (Galium aparine)

- **Profile:** A climbing plant with tiny hook-like hairs on the stems and leaves.
- **Uses:** Used as a lymphatic system tonic and diuretic. Also applied topically for skin ailments such as eczema and psoriasis.

Cloves (Syzygium aromaticum)

- **Profile:** The aromatic flower buds of a tree in the family Myrtaceae.
- **Uses:** Widely used as a spice. In herbal medicine, cloves are known for their analgesic properties, particularly for dental pain, and their digestive and antimicrobial benefits.

Cnidium (Cnidium monnieri)

- **Profile:** A plant used in traditional Chinese medicine.
- **Uses:** The seeds treat skin conditions like eczema and rashes. Also used to improve libido and treat erectile dysfunction.

Coleus Forskohlii

- **Profile:** A tropical perennial plant.
- **Uses:** The root extract, known as forskolin, is used to increase levels of cyclic AMP in the body, which can promote weight loss, support cardiovascular health, and improve eye health.

Coltsfoot (Tussilago farfara)

- **Profile:** A plant with yellow flowers resembling small dandelions.
- **Uses:** Used as a traditional remedy for cough and sore throat. It's an expectorant, helping to clear mucus from the lungs.

Columbine (Aquilegia spp.)

- **Profile:** A flowering plant with distinctive spurred flowers.
- **Uses:** Historically used in small amounts for its astringent and diuretic properties, though not commonly used today due to potential toxicity.

Comfrey (Symphytum officinale)

- **Profile:** A perennial herb with broad, hairy leaves and bell-shaped flowers.
- **Uses:** Used topically for its wound-healing properties to treat bruises, sprains, and bone fractures. It is not recommended for internal use due to potential toxicity.

Common Mallow (Malva sylvestris)

- **Profile:** A plant with soft, round leaves and pink flowers.
- **Uses:** Due to their mucilage content, the leaves and flowers are used for their soothing properties, especially for the throat and digestive system.

Coriander (Coriandrum sativum)

- **Profile:** Commonly known for its seeds (coriander) and leaves (cilantro).
- **Uses:** The seeds are used as a spice and for digestive issues, while the leaves are popular in culinary dishes. Coriander has antibacterial properties and may aid in blood sugar regulation.

Cornflower (Centaurea cyanus)

- **Profile:** A plant with bright blue flowers or a bachelor's button.
- **Uses:** Used in traditional medicine for its anti-inflammatory properties and as a treatment for eye discomfort.

Couch Grass (Elymus repens)

- **Profile:** A persistent weed also known as quackgrass.
- **Uses:** The rhizomes are used for their diuretic properties, helping to flush out the urinary tract and treat bladder infections.

Cowslip (Primula veris)

- **Profile:** A flowering plant with clusters of yellow flowers.
- **Uses:** Used for its soothing and expectorant properties in treating respiratory conditions like bronchitis and asthma.

Crampbark (Viburnum opulus)

- **Profile:** A shrub with white flowers and red berries.
- **Uses:** As the name suggests, it relieves cramps, including menstrual cramps and muscle spasms. Also used for its soothing and anti-inflammatory properties.

Cranesbill (Geranium spp.)

- **Profile:** Also known as wild geranium or alum root.
- **Uses:** The root is used for its astringent properties to treat diarrhea and internal bleeding.

Creosote Bush (Larrea tridentata)

- **Profile:** A shrub native to the deserts of the Southwestern U.S. and Mexico.
- **Uses:** Traditionally used for various ailments, including inflammation, arthritis, and digestive issues. Known for its strong antiseptic properties.

Culver's Root (Veronicastrum virginicum)

- **Profile:** A tall, native North American perennial herb.
- **Uses:** Traditionally used as a laxative and to stimulate liver function. It has also been used to treat digestive disorders and as a tonic to purify the blood.

Cumin (Cuminum cyminum)

- **Profile:** A flowering plant whose seeds are used as a spice, especially in Middle Eastern and Indian cuisines.
- **Uses:** Cumin aids digestion, improves immunity, and provides iron. It also has antiseptic properties and is used in remedies for colds and flu.

Curry Leaves (Murraya koenigii)

- **Profile:** Aromatic leaves from the curry tree are commonly used in Indian and Sri Lankan cooking.
- **Uses:** Besides culinary uses, curry leaves are believed to have anti-diabetic properties, aid digestion, and promote hair growth.

Curry Powder

- **Profile:** A blend of spices typically includes turmeric, coriander, cumin, fenugreek, and chili peppers.
- **Uses:** Used primarily for flavor in cooking, the individual spices in curry powder have various health benefits, including anti-inflammatory and antioxidant properties.

HERBS D - E: PROFILES AND USES

Daikon (Raphanus sativus var. longipinnatus)

- **Profile:** A mild-flavored winter radish commonly found in East Asian cuisine.
- **Uses:** Daikon is eaten for its digestive benefits and is believed to have detoxifying properties. It's rich in vitamins and minerals and can aid digestion and respiratory health.

Damiana (Turnera diffusa)

- **Profile:** A small shrub native to Southern Texas, Mexico, Central and South America, known for its aromatic leaves.
- **Uses:** Traditionally used as an aphrodisiac, Damiana also acts as a mood enhancer and a mild antidepressant. It's often taken to relieve anxiety, nervousness, and mild depression.

Dandelion (Taraxacum officinale)

- **Profile:** Often regarded as a weed, dandelion is a highly nutritious plant with bright yellow flowers.
- **Uses:** The leaves are used as a diuretic, the roots are used for liver detoxification, and the flowers are used in making dandelion wine. Rich in vitamins and minerals, it's also used to aid digestion and skin health.

Daisy (Bellis perennis)

- **Profile:** A common lawn weed with a familiar white and yellow flower.
- **Uses:** Traditionally used for its anti-inflammatory properties and to treat minor wounds.

Dang Shen (Codonopsis pilosula)

- **Profile:** A plant used in traditional Chinese medicine, often as a substitute for ginseng.
- **Uses:** Used to boost the immune system, increase stamina and endurance, and treat digestive issues.

Devil's Bit Scabious (Succisa pratensis)

- **Profile:** A flowering plant with purple-blue flowers.
- **Uses:** Traditionally used for skin conditions, coughs, and as an anti-inflammatory.

Devil's Claw (Harpagophytum procumbens)

- **Profile:** A plant native to South Africa, known for its hook-like fruit.
- **Uses:** The root is used for its anti-inflammatory and analgesic properties, making it a popular treatment for arthritis, rheumatism, and back pain.

Dichroa (Dichroa febrifuga)

- **Profile:** An evergreen shrub with hydrangea-like flowers.
- **Uses:** Used in traditional Chinese medicine for its antimalarial properties.

Dill (Anethum graveolens)

- **Profile:** An aromatic herb with feathery leaves commonly used in cooking.
- **Uses:** Dill is known for its digestive and carminative properties. It's used to treat indigestion, flatulence, and colic in babies. The seeds are also used for their calming effect and to aid sleep.

Dog Grass (Elymus repens)

- **Profile:** Also known as quackgrass, a common garden weed.
- **Uses:** The roots are used for their diuretic and soothing urinary properties.

Dong Quai (Angelica sinensis)

- **Profile:** A traditional Chinese medicinal herb called "female ginseng."
- **Uses:** Widely used to treat menstrual cramps, regulate menstrual cycles, and alleviate menopausal symptoms. It's also believed to improve blood circulation.

Duckweed (Lemnoideae)

- **Profile:** Small, floating aquatic plants.
- **Uses:** Used for its high protein content and fast growth, often in animal feed. In traditional medicine, it's used for its anti-inflammatory properties.

Dwarf Milkwort (Polygala amara)

- **Profile:** A small plant with blue flowers.
- **Uses:** Used in traditional medicine for its expectorant and tonic properties.

Echinacea Purpurea (Purple Coneflower)

- **Profile:** A popular perennial herb native to North America, known for its distinctive purple flowers.
- **Uses:** Widely used to boost the immune system and reduce the symptoms of colds, flu, and other infections. Echinacea is also used topically for wounds and skin problems due to its anti-inflammatory properties.

Elderberry (Sambucus nigra)

- **Profile:** A plant bearing clusters of small black or dark blue berries.
- **Uses:** Elderberry is renowned for its immune-boosting properties. It's commonly used in syrups, teas, and supplements to prevent or alleviate cold and flu symptoms. The berries are also high in antioxidants and vitamins.

Elecampane (Inula helenium)

- **Profile:** A tall perennial plant with yellow flowers and a large rhizome.
- **Uses:** Used for its expectorant and anti-inflammatory properties, particularly for treating respiratory conditions like bronchitis and asthma.

Eleuthero (Eleutherococcus senticosus)

- **Profile:** Also known as Siberian ginseng, though not a true ginseng.
- **Uses:** Used as an adaptogen to increase stress resistance and boost energy and immune function.

Elm Bark (Ulmus spp.)

- **Profile:** The inner bark of elm trees.
- **Uses:** Used for its soothing, mucilaginous properties in treating sore throats, coughs, and digestive issues.

English Ivy (Hedera helix)

- **Profile:** A common climbing vine.
- **Uses:** The leaves treat respiratory tract congestion due to their expectorant properties.

Ephedra (Ephedra sinica)

- **Profile:** A plant known for its stimulant properties.
- **Uses:** Used to treat colds, flu, and asthma. Due to safety concerns, products containing ephedra alkaloids are banned in the U.S.

Eucalyptus (Eucalyptus spp.)

- **Profile:** A fast-growing tree native to Australia, known for its aromatic leaves.
- **Uses:** Eucalyptus leaves and oil relieves coughs, colds, and congestion. It's also applied topically for pain relief and as an antiseptic. The scent of eucalyptus oil is popular in aromatherapy for its refreshing and invigorating properties.

Eyebright (Euphrasia officinalis)

- **Profile:** A small herb bearing white flowers with purple streaks, commonly found in meadows and grassy areas.
- **Uses:** Traditionally used to relieve eye irritations such as conjunctivitis and eyestrain. Eyebright is often used in eye drops and compresses for its anti-inflammatory and astringent properties.

Evening Primrose Oil (Oenothera biennis)

- **Profile:** Derived from the evening primrose plant's seeds, this oil is rich in omega-6 fatty acids.
- **Uses:** Evening primrose oil is widely used for its potential to ease menstrual and menopausal symptoms, including PMS and hot flashes. It's also used for skin conditions like eczema and psoriasis, improving overall skin health. Its anti-inflammatory properties make it beneficial for conditions like rheumatoid arthritis.

HERBS F - G: PROFILES AND USES

False Unicorn (Chamaelirium luteum)

- **Profile:** A perennial herb with small white flowers.
- **Uses:** Traditionally used for reproductive health, including promoting fertility and treating menstrual disorders.

Fennel (Foeniculum vulgare)

- **Profile:** A highly aromatic and flavorful herb with feathery leaves and yellow flowers. Both the bulb and seeds are used.
- **Uses:** Fennel seeds are known for their digestive and carminative properties, helping to relieve gas, bloating, and stomach cramps. It's also used for its mild diuretic effect and to improve milk supply in breastfeeding mothers.

Fenugreek (Trigonella foenum-graecum)

- **Profile:** An annual plant with light green leaves and small white flowers, known for its cuboid-shaped, yellow-to-amber colored seeds.
- **Uses:** Widely used to enhance libido and increase testosterone levels. Fenugreek is also popular for its ability to improve blood sugar control, enhance lactation, and soothe skin inflammation.

Feverfew (Tanacetum parthenium)

- **Profile:** A medicinal plant with daisy-like flowers native to Eurasia.
- **Uses:** Traditionally used for treating fevers, headaches, and particularly migraines. It's also used as an anti-inflammatory for joint pains and arthritis.

Five Finger Grass (Potentilla reptans)

- **Profile:** Also known as cinquefoil, it's a low-growing plant with yellow flowers.
- **Uses:** Traditionally used for its astringent properties and for treating gastrointestinal issues.

Flaxseed Oil (Linum usitatissimum)

- **Profile:** Oil extracted from the seeds of the flax plant, high in omega-3 fatty acids.
- **Uses:** Flaxseed oil is used for its heart-healthy benefits, including lowering cholesterol and blood pressure. It's also beneficial for skin health, reducing inflammation, and aiding digestive health.

Fo-Ti Root (Polygonum multiflorum)

- **Profile:** A traditional Chinese herb also known as He Shou Wu.
- **Uses:** Used to treat aging symptoms, increase longevity, improve sexual function, and enhance hair growth. It's also known for its liver and kidney tonic properties.

Fringe Tree (Chionanthus virginicus)

- **Profile:** A tree with fragrant white flowers.
- **Uses:** The bark is used to support liver and gallbladder health and for its mild diuretic properties.

Fumitory (Fumaria officinalis)

- **Profile:** A flowering plant in the poppy family.
- **Uses:** Used for its detoxifying effects, particularly on the liver and gallbladder, and for treating skin conditions.

Galangal (Alpinia galanga)

- **Profile:** A ginger family plant known for its culinary and medicinal uses.
- **Uses:** Used to aid digestion, reduce inflammation, and relieve discomfort from ulcers and stomach pain.

Galla (Rhus chinensis)

- **Profile:** Also known as Chinese gall, it is formed by aphids on the leaves of the Rhus chinensis tree.
- **Uses:** Used traditionally in tanning and traditional medicine to treat diarrhea, excessive sweating, and bleeding.

Ganoderma (Ganoderma lucidum)

- **Profile:** Commonly known as Reishi mushroom, it is a type of medicinal fungus.
- **Uses:** Reishi is used for its immune-boosting properties, stress reduction, and as a liver tonic. Also thought to improve energy levels and cardiovascular health.

Garam Masala

- **Profile:** A blend of ground spices used extensively in Indian cuisine.
- **Uses:** While primarily used for flavouring dishes, the individual spices in garam masala, like cumin, coriander, and cardamom, have digestive and anti-inflammatory properties.

Garcinia Cambogia

- **Profile:** A small, pumpkin-shaped fruit native to Southeast Asia.
- **Uses:** The extract, known as hydroxy citric acid, is popular in weight loss supplements. It's believed to inhibit fat production and suppress appetite.

Garlic (Allium sativum)

- **Profile:** A well-known culinary herb and a medicinal plant.
- **Uses:** Used to reduce cholesterol levels, lower blood pressure, and improve heart health. Garlic has strong antimicrobial properties and is used to boost the immune system.

Gentian (Gentiana lutea)

- **Profile:** A herb with bright blue flowers known for its intensely bitter roots.
- **Uses:** Used as a digestive tonic to stimulate appetite and improve digestive function.

Geranium (Pelargonium spp.)

- **Profile:** A flowering plant with fragrant leaves, often used in essential oils.
- **Uses:** Geranium oil is used for its astringent properties in skincare and to reduce stress and anxiety. It's also used as a natural insect repellent.

Ginger (Zingiber officinale)

- **Profile:** A widely used spice and medicinal herb with a strong, spicy flavour.
- **Uses:** Renowned for its digestive benefits, particularly in treating nausea and vomiting. Also used for its anti-inflammatory properties and to alleviate menstrual pain.

Ginkgo Biloba

- **Profile:** An ancient tree species known for its distinctive fan-shaped leaves.
- **Uses:** Used to improve cognitive function, treat dementia symptoms, and enhance blood circulation. It's also thought to have antioxidant properties.

Ginseng (Panax spp.)

- **Profile:** A medicinal root highly regarded in traditional Chinese medicine.
- **Uses:** Used as an adaptogen to increase energy levels, reduce stress, and improve immune function. Also thought to have anti-aging properties.

Glucosamine

- **Profile:** A natural compound found in cartilage.
- **Uses:** Commonly used in dietary supplements to support joint health and relieve osteoarthritis symptoms.

Goat Willow (Salix caprea)

- **Profile:** Also known as pussy willow, a species of willow with soft, furry catkins.
- **Uses:** The bark is used for its pain-relieving and anti-inflammatory

properties, similar to aspirin.

Goldenseal (Hydrastis canadensis)

- **Profile:** A perennial herb native to North America.
- **Uses:** Used for its antimicrobial properties, particularly for infections in the mucous membranes. Also used as a digestive tonic and immune system enhancer.

Goldthread (Coptis chinensis)

- **Profile:** A plant with yellow, thread-like roots.
- **Uses:** In traditional Chinese medicine, goldthread is known for its anti-inflammatory and antibacterial properties and is often used for digestive health and skin conditions.

Goji Berries (Lycium barbarum)

- **Profile:** A bright red berry from a shrub native to China.
- **Uses:** Consumed for their high nutrient content, antioxidant properties, and potential to improve energy, visual acuity, and overall vitality.

Gotu Kola (Centella asiatica)

- **Profile:** An herbaceous plant used in Ayurvedic and traditional Chinese medicine.
- **Uses:** Known for improving cognitive function, healing skin wounds, and reducing varicose veins and cellulite.

Great Burnet (Sanguisorba officinalis)

- **Profile:** A plant with dark red flowers, traditionally used in herbal medicine.
- **Uses:** Used for its astringent properties to treat gastrointestinal issues and to stop bleeding.

Great Mullein (Verbascum thapsus)

- **Profile:** A tall herb with a dense spike of yellow flowers and large leaves.
- **Uses:** The leaves and flowers are used for their soothing properties on the respiratory system, particularly in treating coughs and bronchitis.

Greater Celandine (Chelidonium majus)

- **Profile:** A herb with yellow flowers and a distinctive orange sap.
- **Uses:** Traditionally used to treat liver disorders and gallbladder issues. The sap is applied topically to remove warts.

Green-lipped mussels (Perna canaliculus)

- **Profile:** A type of mussel native to New Zealand.
- **Uses:** The extract is used in supplements for its anti-inflammatory properties, particularly in treating joint pain and arthritis symptoms.

Green Tea (Camellia sinensis)

- **Profile:** Made from the leaves of the Camellia sinensis plant, known for its antioxidant properties.
- **Uses:** Consumed for its potential to boost metabolism, improve heart health, and lower the risk of certain types of cancer.

Grindelia (Grindelia spp.)

- **Profile:** A plant known for its gum resin is used in medicinal preparations.
- **Uses:** Used as an expectorant for respiratory conditions and a topical remedy for skin irritations.

Guaiac Resin (Guaiacum officinale)

- **Profile:** A resin extracted from the wood of the Guaiacum plant.
- **Uses:** Traditionally used as a remedy for syphilis rheumatism and as a laxative. Also used in diagnostic tests for blood in stool.

Guapi Bark (Clathrotropis brachypetala)

- **Profile:** Bark from the Guapi tree, native to South America.
- **Uses:** Used in traditional medicine for its anti-inflammatory properties and to treat skin conditions and wounds.

Guarana (Paullinia cupana)

- **Profile:** A plant native to the Amazon basin, known for its seeds with more caffeine than coffee beans.
- **Uses:** Used as a stimulant to reduce mental and physical fatigue. Also used in weight loss supplements and to enhance athletic performance.

Guava (Psidium guajava)

- **Profile:** A tropical fruit rich in vitamins and antioxidants.
- **Uses:** The fruit is eaten for its nutritional value. Guava leaves are used in traditional medicine to treat diarrhea, lower blood sugar levels, and as an antibacterial agent.

Gum Asafetida (Ferula asafoetida)

- **Profile:** The dried sap of the Ferula plant with a strong, pungent smell.
- **Uses:** Used in cooking, particularly in Indian cuisine, and medicinally for its digestive properties as a remedy for flatulence and irritable bowel syndrome.

Gum Plant (Grindelia spp.)

- **Profile:** A genus of plants known for their sticky, resinous flower buds.
- **Uses:** Traditionally used to treat bronchial conditions and as a natural expectorant. Also used topically for skin irritations and rashes.

Gum Tragacanth (Astragalus gummifer)

- **Profile:** A thorny shrub that produces a natural gum.
- **Uses:** The gum is used in pharmaceuticals and foods as a stabilizer. It has been used in traditional medicine for its soothing properties.

Gymnema Sylvestre

- **Profile:** A woody climbing shrub native to India and Africa.
- **Uses:** Known for its ability to reduce the absorption of sugar from the intestine and to help regulate blood sugar levels, particularly in diabetes.

HERBS H - J: PROFILES AND USES

Hawthorn Berry (Crataegus spp.)

- **Profile:** A small red berry from the hawthorn shrub, rich in bioflavonoids.
- **Uses:** Hawthorn is primarily used for its cardiovascular benefits. It improves heart health, enhances blood circulation, and manages blood pressure. Also used as a mild sedative and for digestive issues.

Heather (Calluna vulgaris)

- **Profile:** A small shrub with pink or purple flowers commonly found on moors and heaths.
- **Uses:** Used traditionally for urinary conditions, such as kidney stones and bladder infections. Also used for sleep disorders, anxiety, and inflammatory conditions.

Hellebore (Helleborus spp.)

- **Profile:** A genus of flowering plants with beautiful, early-spring blooms.
- **Uses:** Historically used for heart and nervous system conditions. Due to its toxicity, it's rarely used in modern herbal medicine and should be handled carefully.

Hemp (Cannabis sativa)

- **Profile:** A variety of the Cannabis sativa plant species grown specifically for industrial uses of its derived products.
- **Uses:** Hemp seeds are rich in omega-3 and omega-6 fatty acids and are used for nutritional value. Hemp oil is used for skin conditions like eczema and to reduce inflammation. CBD oil, derived from hemp, is used for pain relief, anxiety, and as a sleep aid.

Henbane (Hyoscyamus niger)

- **Profile:** A poisonous plant historically used in traditional medicine.
- **Uses:** Used in the past for its soothing and antispasmodic effects, but due to its high toxicity, it is no longer commonly used and is considered dangerous.

Henna (Lawsonia inermis)

- **Profile:** A plant known for its reddish-brown dye used in body art.
- **Uses:** The leaves are used to dye hair and skin. The dye has also been used traditionally to cool the skin and as an anti-fungal.

Hepatica (Hepatica nobilis)

- **Profile:** A small plant with purple, blue, or white flowers and round-lobed leaves.
- **Uses:** Traditionally used as an astringent for liver and gallbladder disorders, but little evidence supports these uses.

Hibiscus (Hibiscus sabdariffa)

- **Profile:** A flowering plant known for its large, colourful flowers.
- **Uses:** Hibiscus tea, made from the plant's calyces, is consumed for its potential to lower blood pressure, its diuretic properties, and its high vitamin C content. Also used for liver health and as a mild laxative.

Holly (Ilex spp.)

- **Profile:** A widely recognized plant, especially around Christmas, known for its distinctive red berries and glossy, pointed leaves.
- **Uses:** While often used for decoration, some species of holly, like Yerba Mate (Ilex paraguariensis), are used for their stimulating properties to enhance alertness and mental focus.

Hoodia Gordonii

- **Profile:** A succulent Kalahari Desert plant known for its appetite-suppressant properties.
- **Uses:** Used for weight loss to help curb hunger and appetite, although scientific evidence supporting its effectiveness is limited.

Hops (Humulus lupulus)

- **Profile:** Known for their use in brewing beer, hops are soothing.
- **Uses:** Used to treat insomnia, anxiety, and restlessness. Also has estrogen-like properties and is used for symptoms of menopause.

Horehound (Marrubium vulgare)

- **Profile:** A herb with white, woolly leaves and a bitter taste.
- **Uses:** Traditionally used as an expectorant to treat coughs and colds. Also used for digestive disorders due to its bitter principles.

Horny Goat Weed (Epimedium spp.)

- **Profile:** A herbaceous plant native to China, known for its heart-shaped leaves.
- **Uses:** Traditionally used as an aphrodisiac and to treat erectile dysfunction. Also believed to improve bone health, protect the heart, and reduce symptoms of menopause.

Horse Chestnut (Aesculus hippocastanum)

- **Profile:** A tree known for its large, inedible nuts, or "conkers."
- **Uses:** The extract from horse chestnut seeds treats chronic venous insufficiency, reducing leg swelling and improving blood flow. Also used for hemorrhoids and varicose veins.

Horseradish (Armoracia rusticana)

- **Profile:** A plant known for its spicy root, commonly used as a condiment.
- **Uses:** Used for its potential to clear sinuses and treat urinary tract infections. Rich in vitamin C and believed to have antibacterial properties.

Horsetail (Equisetum arvense)

- **Profile:** A perennial fern-like plant, rich in silica.
- **Uses:** Horsetail is used to improve bone health, for hair and nail strength, and as a mild diuretic. Also applied topically to heal wounds and burns.

Humulus (Humulus lupulus)

- **Profile:** Commonly known as hops, these are the flowers of the hop plant, primarily used in brewing beer.
- **Uses:** Medicinally, hops are used for their sedative effects to treat insomnia, anxiety, and restlessness. Also used for digestive issues due to

their bitter compounds.

Hydrangea (Hydrangea spp.)

- **Profile:** A genus of ornamental plants with large flower heads.
- **Uses:** The root is used for its diuretic properties and to treat kidney stones and bladder infections.

Hyssop (Hyssopus officinalis)

- **Profile:** An aromatic herb used in cooking and herbal medicine.
- **Uses:** Used for its expectorant properties to treat respiratory conditions and as an antiseptic. Also used for digestion and muscle aches.

Ignatia (Strychnos ignatii)

- **Profile:** Also known as Ignatius bean, it's derived from the seeds of the Strychnos gigantic tree in Southeast Asia.
- **Uses:** In homeopathy, Ignatia is used to treat a range of psychological issues like anxiety, depression, and stress. It's known for addressing emotional upheavals and grief.

Iceland Moss (Cetraria islandica)

- **Profile:** A lichen found in the mountainous regions of the Northern Hemisphere.
- **Uses:** Used for its mucilaginous properties, which can soothe irritated mucous membranes in the throat and stomach. Also used as a nutritive tonic due to its polysaccharide content.

Irish Moss (Chondrus crispus)

- **Profile:** A type of red algae or seaweed that grows along the Atlantic coastlines.
- **Uses:** Irish moss is rich in nutrients and is used as a thickener and emulsifier in foods. Medicinally, it's used for its soothing properties, particularly respiratory and digestive health.

Jamaica Dogwood (Piscidia piscipula)

- **Profile:** A tree found in the West Indies and parts of the Americas.
- **Uses:** Used for its sedative, analgesic, and antispasmodic properties. Traditionally used to treat nervous tension, insomnia, and pain, particularly migraine and menstrual cramps.

Jamaica Ginger (Zingiber officinale)

- **Profile:** The same ginger plant is known for its culinary uses, but this refers specifically to the variety grown in Jamaica.
- **Uses:** Used for its anti-inflammatory, digestive, and anti-nausea properties. It is also used to alleviate arthritis pain and boost circulation.

Juniper (Juniperus communis)

- **Profile:** An evergreen shrub with needle-like leaves and blue-black berries.
- **Uses:** Juniper berries are used for their diuretic properties and to treat urinary tract infections and kidney stones. They also have anti-inflammatory and antiseptic effects, making them useful in treating rheumatism and arthritis.

HERBS K - L: PROFILES AND USES

Kale (Brassica oleracea var. sabellica)

- **Profile:** A type of cabbage with green or purple leaves known for its nutritional value.
- **Uses:** Consumed for its high levels of vitamins, minerals, and antioxidants. Kale is also believed to aid in cardiovascular and digestive health.

Kava Kava (Piper methysticum)

- **Profile:** A plant native to the South Pacific islands, known for its psychoactive properties.
- **Uses:** Kava is consumed for its soothing effects, primarily for reducing anxiety and promoting relaxation. It is traditionally used in social and ceremonial settings.

Kelp (Laminariales spp.)

- **Profile:** Large brown algae seaweeds that make up the order Laminariales.
- **Uses:** Kelp is a natural iodine source commonly used to support thyroid function. It's also rich in minerals and is used as a nutritional supplement.

Khella (Ammi visnaga)

- **Profile:** A plant native to the Mediterranean region.
- **Uses:** The active compound khellin has been used to treat asthma and coronary spasms. It's also used as a diuretic and for kidney stone prevention.

Kino (Pterocarpus marsupium)

- **Profile:** A tree found in India, known for its heartwood that exudes a dark gum known as kino.
- **Uses:** The gum is used traditionally to treat diarrhea and other gastrointestinal issues. It's also used in Ayurvedic medicine for its anti-diabetic properties and to promote skin healing.

Knotgrass (Polygonum aviculare)

- **Profile:** A common weed with a sprawling habit and tiny flowers.
- **Uses:** Traditionally used for respiratory ailments, as a diuretic, and for its anti-inflammatory properties.

Kudzu (Pueraria lobata)

- **Profile:** A vine native to Asia, known for its rapid growth and use in traditional Chinese medicine.
- **Uses:** Used to treat alcoholism, menopause symptoms, diabetes, fever, and heart disease, although more research is needed to support these uses fully.

Lady's Mantle (Alchemilla vulgaris)

- **Profile:** A perennial plant with fan-shaped leaves and tiny yellowish-green flowers.
- **Uses:** Used traditionally for menstrual and menopausal disorders due to its astringent properties. Also used for gastrointestinal issues.

Lady's Slipper (Cypripedium spp.)

- **Profile:** A wild orchid known for its unique, slipper-shaped flowers.
- **Uses:** Historically used as a sedative and for nervous system conditions. Due to its rarity, it's not commonly used today and is protected in many areas.

Lamb's Quarters (Chenopodium album)

- **Profile:** A common garden weed with edible leaves.
- **Uses:** The leaves are high in vitamins and minerals and can be eaten as a nutritious vegetable. Traditionally used as an anti-inflammatory and to treat digestive issues.

Lavender (Lavandula spp.)

- **Profile:** A fragrant herb known for its purple flowers and soothing aroma.
- **Uses:** Widely used in aromatherapy for relaxation and stress relief. Topically, it's applied for its antiseptic and anti-inflammatory properties, helping to soothe and heal minor burns, insect bites, and skin irritations. Also used in teas to aid sleep and alleviate digestive issues.

Lemon Balm (Melissa officinalis)

- **Profile:** A perennial herb in the mint family with a lemony scent and flavor.
- **Uses:** Lemon balm is used for its calming effect to relieve anxiety, insomnia, and restlessness. It's also known for improving digestion and relieving symptoms of indigestion.

Lemongrass (Cymbopogon)

- **Profile:** A tall, stalky plant with a fresh, lemony aroma and a citrus flavor.
- **Uses:** In culinary, it's used in teas and flavoring. Medicinally, lemongrass is used for its analgesic properties to relieve pain and reduce fever. It also has antifungal and antibacterial properties.

Lemon Myrtle (Backhousia citriodora)

- **Profile:** An Australian native plant known for its strong lemon scent.
- **Uses:** Used in cooking for its lemony flavor. It's used for its antimicrobial and antifungal properties, particularly in treating oral and skin infections. Also used in aromatherapy for relaxation.

Licorice Root (Glycyrrhiza glabra)

- **Profile:** A root used for its sweet flavor and various medicinal properties.
- **Uses:** Traditionally used to soothe gastrointestinal problems, such as acid reflux, ulcers, and indigestion. It also has anti-inflammatory and immune-boosting properties. However, excessive consumption can lead to adverse effects.

Life Root (Senecio aureus)

- **Profile:** A perennial herb with yellow flowers.
- **Uses:** Traditionally used for women's health issues such as irregular menstruation and to ease childbirth.

Lime (Citrus aurantiifolia)

- **Profile:** A citrus fruit known for its acidic juice and fragrant peel.
- **Uses:** Besides culinary uses, lime is used for its vitamin C content and potential benefits in improving digestion, skin health, and preventing infections. Lime juice and oil are also used in aromatherapy.

Linden (Tilia spp.)

- **Profile:** Trees are known for their fragrant flowers and heart-shaped leaves.
- **Uses:** Linden flowers are used in teas for their calming effect and to help reduce mild anxiety. Also used for reducing cold symptoms and promoting relaxation.

Lobelia (Lobelia inflata)

- **Profile:** Also known as Indian tobacco, it's a plant with small blue flowers.
- **Uses:** Historically used to treat respiratory conditions like asthma and bronchitis. It acts as a bronchodilator and expectorant. Due to its potency, it should be used under professional guidance.

Loquat (Eriobotrya japonica)

- **Profile:** A fruit tree native to China, known for its yellow, tangy-sweet fruit.
- **Uses:** The loquat fruit is eaten for its nutritional value. Due to their anti-

inflammatory properties, Loquat leaves are used in traditional medicine for respiratory ailments, including coughs and asthma.

Lovage (Levisticum officinale)

- **Profile:** A perennial plant resembling celery with a strong, aromatic flavour.
- **Uses:** Used for its diuretic properties and to treat digestive issues. Also used for menstrual and urinary tract problems.

Lungwort (Pulmonaria officinalis)

- **Profile:** A perennial plant with spotted leaves and clusters of blue, pink, or white flowers.
- **Uses:** Traditionally used for respiratory conditions such as coughs and bronchitis due to its mucilage content. It's also used for its soothing and anti-inflammatory properties.

Lycopene

- **Profile:** A bright red carotenoid pigment in tomatoes and other red fruits and vegetables.
- **Uses:** Known for its antioxidant properties, lycopene is consumed to reduce the risk of cancer and heart disease. It's also used for its potential benefits in protecting skin from damage by UV light.

Lycopodium (Lycopodium clavatum)

- **Profile:** Also known as clubmoss, this perennial plant has small, scale-like leaves.
- **Uses:** Lycopodium is used for digestive disorders and liver complaints and as a cognitive enhancer in homeopathy. It is also used for skin conditions like eczema and psoriasis.

HERBS M - O: PROFILES AND USES

Maca (Lepidium meyenii)

- **Profile:** A Peruvian root vegetable known for its nutrient-rich profile.
- **Uses:** Often consumed as a supplement for its ability to increase libido, enhance energy and endurance, and balance hormones. It's also believed to improve fertility and reduce menopausal symptoms.

Macadamia (Macadamia spp.)

- **Profile:** A genus of trees native to Australia, known for their rich, buttery-tasting nuts.
- **Uses:** The nuts are highly nutritious and rich in healthy fats, vitamins, and minerals. They're consumed for their potential to improve heart health, aid weight management, and as an antioxidant source.

Mace (Myristica fragrans)

- **Profile:** The aromatic spice is made from the dried reddish seed covering of the nutmeg.
- **Uses:** Used for flavouring in cooking. In herbal medicine, it's used for its digestive properties, stimulating appetite, and relieving nausea and vomiting.

Madder (Rubia tinctorum)

- **Profile:** A plant historically used for the red dye obtained from its roots.
- **Uses:** Traditionally used to treat kidney and urinary disorders, although not commonly used in modern herbal medicine.

Magnolia (Magnolia officinalis)

- **Profile:** A large genus of flowering plants.
- **Uses:** Magnolia bark is used in traditional Chinese medicine for stress relief and to help with sleep. It's also used for digestive disorders and as an anti-inflammatory.

Malabar Nut (Justicia adhatoda)

- **Profile:** A medicinal plant in Asia known for its bronchodilator effect.
- **Uses:** Used to treat respiratory conditions like asthma and bronchitis. It acts as an expectorant and helps to relieve cough.

Mandrake (Mandragora officinarum)

- **Profile:** A plant known for its large root that resembles the human form.
- **Uses:** Traditionally used as an anesthetic and a sleep aid due to its hallucinogenic and sedative properties. Its use is largely historical due to toxicity and legal issues.

Marigold (Calendula officinalis)

- **Profile:** A bright orange-yellow flowering plant.
- **Uses:** Widely used in topical skin applications. It helps in wound healing, reducing inflammation, and soothing irritated skin. Also used as an antifungal and antibacterial agent.

Maritime Pine Bark (Pinus pinaster)

- **Profile:** The bark from a species of pine native to the Mediterranean region.
- **Uses:** The extract, known as pycnogenol, is used for its antioxidant properties. It's used to improve circulation, reduce inflammation, and treat allergies.

Marjoram (Origanum majorana)

- **Profile:** A sweet, pine, and citrus-flavoured herb in the mint family.
- **Uses:** In herbal medicine, marjoram is used for its calming properties, to ease digestion, to relieve menstrual cramps, and as a general tonic for the nervous system.

Marshmallow (Althaea officinalis)

- **Profile:** A perennial herb with soft, velvety leaves.
- **Uses:** Known for its mucilage content, marshmallow root is used to soothe mucous membranes, relieve irritation of the respiratory and digestive tracts, and in skin care.

Marsh Woundwort (Stachys palustris)

- **Profile:** A plant with purple flowers found in wetlands and moist areas.
- **Uses:** Traditionally used for its antiseptic properties and to treat wounds.

Masterwort (Peucedanum ostruthium)

- **Profile:** A perennial herb in the carrot family with white or pinkish flowers.
- **Uses:** Used in traditional European herbal medicine for digestive issues, respiratory problems, and to stimulate circulation.

Meadowsweet (Filipendula ulmaria)

- **Profile:** A perennial herb with fragrant, creamy-white flowers.
- **Uses:** It contains salicylates and is used for its pain-relieving and anti-inflammatory effects. Traditionally used to treat fevers, colds, and acid indigestion.

Mezereum (Daphne mezereum)

- **Profile:** A species of Daphne with pink and purple flowers and red berries.
- **Uses:** Used in homeopathy for skin conditions like eczema and rheumatic pain. The plant is highly toxic and should be used only under professional guidance.

Milk Thistle (Silybum marianum)

- **Profile:** A flowering herb with distinctive purple flowers and white veins.
- **Uses:** Primarily used for liver health, including liver detoxification and treatment of liver diseases. It's also used for gallbladder disorders and to protect against toxins.

Milkweed (Asclepias spp.)

- **Profile:** A group of plants known for their milky sap and attractive flowers.
- **Uses:** While some species are toxic, others have been used in traditional medicine to treat warts and as a diuretic. It's also a crucial plant for monarch butterflies.

Mint (Mentha spp.)

- **Profile:** A popular herb known for its aromatic leaves.
- **Uses:** Widely used for digestive issues, including irritable bowel syndrome (IBS), nausea, and indigestion. Also used in aromatherapy for its refresh-

ing and cooling effect.

Mistletoe (Viscum album)

- **Profile:** A parasitic plant known for its use in traditional winter celebrations.
- **Uses:** Used in herbal medicine for its cardiovascular properties. Also studied for its potential anti-cancer effects.

Moringa Oleifera

- **Profile:** A fast-growing, drought-resistant tree known as the drumstick tree.
- **Uses:** The leaves are highly nutritious and boost energy levels, reduce inflammation, lower cholesterol, and help control blood sugar.

Motherwort (Leonurus cardiaca)

- **Profile:** A herb in the mint family with a long history of medicinal use.
- **Uses:** Used to treat heart conditions, anxiety, and menstrual discomfort. It has calming properties and is used to support women's reproductive health.

Mugwort (Artemisia vulgaris)

- **Profile:** A plant with a strong aroma, part of the daisy family.
- **Uses:** Used for its digestive and soothing properties. Also used as a dream herb to stimulate vivid dreams and for menstrual irregularities.

Muira Puama (Ptychopetalum olacoides)

- **Profile:** A small tree native to the Amazon rainforest.
- **Uses:** Traditionally used as an aphrodisiac and nerve tonic. Also believed to treat sexual dysfunction, increase libido, and improve cognitive function.

Mullein (Verbascum thapsus)

- **Profile:** A plant with soft, woolly leaves and tall flower spikes.
- **Uses:** The leaves and flowers are used for their soothing effect on the respiratory system, treating coughs, bronchitis, and asthma. Also used topically for skin irritations.

Musk-Root (Nardostachys jatamansi)

- **Profile:** A flowering plant of the Valerian family, known for its aromatic rhizome.
- **Uses:** Used as a soothing agent, similar to valerian. Also used traditionally to treat insomnia and anxiety.

Mustard Seeds (Brassica spp.)

- **Profile:** Small round mustard plant seeds used as a spice.
- **Uses:** In herbal medicine, mustard seeds are used for their warming and circulatory-stimulating properties. Used in plasters to relieve muscle pain, rheumatism, and arthritic pain.

Myrrh (Commiphora myrrha)

- **Profile:** A resin obtained from the myrrh tree.
- **Uses:** Used for its powerful antiseptic and anti-inflammatory properties. Commonly used in oral hygiene products and for treating mouth ulcers,

sore throats, and gum diseases. Also used in aromatherapy for relaxation and meditation.

Nasturtium (Tropaeolum majus)

- **Profile:** An ornamental plant with bright, trumpet-shaped flowers and rounded leaves.
- **Uses:** The leaves and flowers are edible and contain high levels of vitamin C. Medicinally, nasturtium is used for its natural antibiotic properties and to treat respiratory infections.

Neem (Azadirachta indica)

- **Profile:** A tree native to the Indian subcontinent, known for its medicinal properties.
- **Uses:** Neem leaves and oil are used for their antiseptic, antifungal, and anti-inflammatory properties. Commonly used in skin care for treating acne and eczema, as a natural insecticide, and in dental care products. Also used in traditional medicine for its detoxifying benefits and to control blood sugar levels.

Nettle (Urtica dioica)

- **Profile:** A perennial herbaceous plant, often regarded as a weed but known for its nutritional and medicinal properties.
- **Uses:** Nettle treats allergies, particularly hay fever, due to its natural antihistamine properties. It's also used for its diuretic properties, to alleviate arthritis symptoms, and as a nutritive tonic rich in minerals.

Night Blooming Cereus (Selenicereus grandiflorus)

- **Profile:** A cactus with large, fragrant flowers that open at night.
- **Uses:** Traditionally used to treat heart palpitations and as a mild sedative. Also used in small doses to treat nervousness and insomnia.

Northern Dock (Rumex longifolius)

- **Profile:** A plant species known for its long leaves and ability to thrive in northern climates.
- **Uses:** While not as commonly used as other docks, like Yellow Dock, it has been used in herbal medicine for its astringent and purgative properties.

Nutmeg (Myristica fragrans)

- **Profile:** A spice made from the seed of the nutmeg tree, native to Indonesia.
- **Uses:** Nutmeg is used in small quantities in cooking for its warm, spicy flavour. Medicinally, it's used for its digestive properties and relieves pain, such as toothaches and muscle pain. It also has soothing properties when used in larger doses but should be used with caution due to its psychoactive effects at high doses.

Oak (Quercus spp.)

- **Profile:** A genus of trees known for their strength and longevity.
- **Uses:** The bark is traditionally used for its astringent properties to treat diarrhea and inflammation. Oak galls are used in tanning and for medicinal purposes.

Oakmoss (Evernia prunastri)

- **Profile:** A species of lichen used in perfumery and traditional medicine.
- **Uses:** Used in aromatherapy for its calming scent. Traditionally used for its antiseptic and antimicrobial properties.

Oat Straw (Avena sativa)

- **Profile:** The green stem of the oat plant is harvested when the seed is at its milky stage.
- **Uses:** Used to support nervous system health, reduce anxiety, and improve sleep. Also known for its benefits to skin health when used in baths.

Olive Leaf (Olea europaea)

- **Profile:** Derived from the leaves of the olive tree, distinct from the well-known olive oil.
- **Uses:** Olive leaf extract is used for its antioxidant, antihypertensive, and anti-inflammatory properties. It's believed to support cardiovascular health, boost the immune system, and help regulate blood sugar levels.

Onions (Allium cepa)

- **Profile:** A widely used vegetable and culinary ingredient in the allium family.
- **Uses:** Beyond their culinary uses, onions are known for their cardiovascular benefits, including lowering blood pressure and reducing the risk of heart disease. They also have anti-inflammatory and antibacterial properties and are used in folk remedies for colds and coughs.

Orach (Atriplex hortensis)

- **Profile:** Also known as saltbush, an edible leafy green.
- **Uses:** Consumed for its high mineral content, especially magnesium. Used in traditional medicine to treat digestive issues due to its mild laxative effect.

Oregano (Origanum vulgare)

- **Profile:** A fragrant herb commonly used in Mediterranean and Mexican cuisine.
- **Uses:** Oregano has potent antibacterial and antifungal properties. It treats respiratory tract disorders, gastrointestinal disorders, menstrual cramps, and urinary tract infections. Oregano oil is particularly known for its antimicrobial and antioxidant properties.

Oregon Grape (Mahonia aquifolium)

- **Profile:** A plant with holly-like leaves and yellow flowers that develop into purple berries.
- **Uses:** The root and bark are used for their antimicrobial properties, primarily to treat skin conditions and support liver function.

HERBS P: PROFILES AND USES

Panax Ginseng

- **Profile:** A slow-growing plant with fleshy roots, regarded as one of the most important herbs in traditional Chinese medicine.
- **Uses:** Used as an adaptogen to reduce stress, improve stamina and concentration, and boost the immune system.

Paneer Dodi (Withania coagulans)

- **Profile:** A plant used in Ayurvedic medicine, also known for its use in making vegetable rennet.
- **Uses:** Used traditionally to treat diabetes and for its diuretic effect.

Parsley (Petroselinum crispum)

- **Profile:** A popular culinary herb used for its fresh, slightly peppery flavour.
- **Uses:** Rich in vitamins and minerals, parsley is used for its diuretic properties, to freshen breath, and to support kidney and urinary health. Also used for its anti-inflammatory and antioxidant properties.

Paprika (Capsicum annuum)

- **Profile:** A spice made from ground sweet and hot peppers.
- **Uses:** Primarily used in cooking for flavour and colour. Paprika contains capsaicin, known for its anti-inflammatory properties, and is rich in antioxidants.

Pasque Flower (Pulsatilla vulgaris)

- **Profile:** A purple flower that blooms around Easter in the Northern Hemisphere.
- **Uses:** Used homeopathically for menstrual pain and as a sedative. It's toxic and should only be used with professional guidance.

Passion Flower (Passiflora incarnata)

- **Profile:** A vine known for its stunning flowers and medicinal properties.
- **Uses:** Used to treat anxiety, insomnia, and nervous disorders. It has a calming effect without impairing cognitive function.

Pau d'Arco (Tabebuia impetiginosa)

- **Profile:** A tree native to South America, known for its pink to purple flowers.
- **Uses:** The bark is used for its antifungal, antiviral, and antibacterial properties. Traditionally used to boost the immune system and to treat a wide range of ailments, from infections to cancer.

Pecan (Carya illinoinensis)

- **Profile:** A type of nut native to Mexico and the southern United States.
- **Uses:** Consumed for their rich, buttery flavour and nutritional benefits, including heart-healthy fats, vitamins, and minerals. Pecans are also

believed to help lower cholesterol levels.

Peanuts (Arachis hypogaea)

- **Profile:** A legume that grows underground, often used as a nut in various cuisines.
- **Uses:** Rich in protein, healthy fats, and various vitamins and minerals. Peanuts are used for their nutritional value and potential cardiovascular benefits.

Pepper (Piper nigrum)

- **Profile:** A flowering vine cultivated for its fruit, known as a peppercorn when dried.
- **Uses:** Used as a spice in cooking. Black pepper has digestive and antioxidant properties and may enhance the absorption of certain nutrients like turmeric.

Peppermint (Mentha × Piperita)

- **Profile:** A hybrid mint, a cross between watermint and spearmint.
- **Uses:** Widely used for its cooling and soothing properties. Peppermint oil is used to relieve digestive issues and headaches and as a decongestant. Also used for its antimicrobial properties.

Periwinkle (Vinca minor)

- **Profile:** A plant with glossy leaves and purple flowers, used ornamentally and medicinally.
- **Uses:** Contains alkaloids used to treat circulatory disorders and cognitive decline. Due to its toxicity, it is not typically used in herbal remedies without professional guidance.

Peruvian Bark (Cinchona spp.)

- **Profile:** A South American tree bark known as the source of quinine.
- **Uses:** Historically used to treat malaria due to its quinine content. Also used for digestive problems and as a pain reliever.

Pheasant's Eye (Adonis vernalis)

- **Profile:** A plant with bright yellow flowers found in Europe and Asia.
- **Uses:** Historically used for heart conditions because of its cardiac glycoside content. It should be used with caution under professional supervision.

Picrorhiza Kurra (Picrorhiza karroo)

- **Profile:** A small perennial herb used in Ayurvedic medicine.
- **Uses:** Used for liver and digestive issues due to its anti-inflammatory and antioxidant properties.

Pine Nuts (Pinus spp.)

- **Profile:** Edible seeds of pine trees.
- **Uses:** Consumed for their rich, sweet, and nutty flavour. Nutritionally beneficial for their high vitamins, minerals, and healthy fat content. Also believed to have appetite-suppressing properties.

Pipsissewa (Chimaphila umbellata)

- **Profile:** A small plant with shiny green leaves and pinkish flowers.
- **Uses:** Traditionally used to treat urinary tract infections and kidney stones due to its diuretic and antiseptic properties.

Pistachios (Pistacia vera)

- **Profile:** A cashew family member known for their distinct green colour and sweet taste.
- **Uses:** Eaten for their nutritional value, including heart-healthy fats, fibre, and antioxidants. It may help improve cholesterol levels and blood sugar control.

Plantain / Common Plantain (Plantago major)

- **Profile:** A common weed with broad leaves and a tall flower spike.
- **Uses:** Used for its wound healing properties. The leaves are used topically to soothe insect bites and stings and internally to treat digestive issues.

Pleurisy Root (Asclepias tuberosa)

- **Profile:** A plant with bright orange flowers, also known as butterfly weed.
- **Uses:** Traditionally used to treat respiratory conditions like pleurisy and bronchitis due to its expectorant properties.

Polypody (Polypodium vulgare)

- **Profile:** A type of fern.
- **Uses:** Historically used for its laxative effects and to treat respiratory conditions.

Pomegranate (Punica granatum)

- **Profile:** A fruit-bearing shrub known for its jewel-like seeds.
- **Uses:** The seeds and juice are consumed for their high antioxidant content, heart health benefits, and potential anti-inflammatory properties. Also used in traditional medicine for digestive and skin health.

Pomegranate Bark

- **Profile:** The bark of the pomegranate tree.
- **Uses:** Used in traditional medicine, mainly for its anthelmintic properties to expel intestinal parasites. However, it must be used with caution due to potential toxicity.

Pokeweed (Phytolacca americana)

- **Profile:** A perennial plant with purplish stems and berries.
- **Uses:** Historically used in small, controlled doses for rheumatism, lymphatic problems, and as an immune stimulant. However, it is highly toxic and not recommended for unguided use.

Poppy Seeds (Papaver somniferum)

- **Profile:** The tiny, edible seeds of the poppy flower.
- **Uses:** Used in cooking for their nutty flavour. Poppy seeds contain linoleic acid and are consumed for their nutritional value. The seeds are non-narcotic and do not contain opium alkaloids found in other parts of the poppy plant.

Prickly Ash Bark (Zanthoxylum americanum)

- **Profile:** A tree with a distinctive spiny bark.
- **Uses:** Used for its circulatory stimulating properties. Traditionally used to treat joint pain, toothache, and digestive issues.

Prickly Pear Cactus (Opuntia spp.)

- **Profile:** A genus of flowering cacti known for their edible fruit.
- **Uses:** The fruit and pads of the prickly pear cactus are consumed for their high fibre content, vitamins, and minerals. Known to help lower blood

sugar levels and improve cholesterol.

Pueraria Mirifica (Kwao Krua)

- **Profile:** A plant native to Thailand, known for its phytoestrogens.
- **Uses:** Used in supplements for menopausal symptom relief, such as hot flashes and mood swings. Also believed to improve skin health and bone strength.

Pumpkin Seeds

- **Profile:** The edible seeds of the pumpkin or certain varieties of squash.
- **Uses:** Consumed for their high magnesium, zinc, and healthy fats content. Pumpkin seeds are believed to benefit heart and prostate health and are used for their anti-inflammatory properties.

Purslane (Portulaca oleracea)

- **Profile:** A succulent leafy plant, often considered a weed.
- **Uses:** Rich in omega-3 fatty acids and antioxidants. Used to treat skin conditions and as a source of nutrients.

Pygeum (Prunus Africana)

- **Profile:** A tree found in Africa, known for its medicinal bark.
- **Uses:** Used to treat symptoms of an enlarged prostate (benign prostatic hyperplasia, BPH) and to promote urinary health.

Psyllium Husk (Plantago ovata)

- **Profile:** The fibrous seed husks of the Plantago ovata plant.
- **Uses:** Widely used as a dietary fibre supplement for improving digestion, relieving constipation, and aiding in weight management. Also beneficial

for heart health and blood sugar control.

Pycnogenol (Pinus pinaster)

- **Profile:** A patented extract of French maritime pine bark.
- **Uses:** Known for its antioxidant properties. Used to improve cardiovascular health, reduce inflammation, and improve skin health. Also used for treating circulation problems, allergies, and asthma.

HERBS Q - R: PROFILES AND USES

Queen's Root (Stillingia sylvatica)

- **Profile:** Also known as Queen's Delight, it's a plant native to the southern United States.
- **Uses:** Traditionally used to support the lymphatic system, for skin conditions, and as a detoxifying agent. Due to its potency, it should be used under professional guidance.

Raspberry (Rubus idaeus)

- **Profile:** A plant known for its delicious, edible red berries.
- **Uses:** Raspberry leaf is used in traditional herbal medicine for its uterine toning properties, particularly during pregnancy and childbirth. The berries are high in nutrients and antioxidants.

Raspberry Leaf (Rubus idaeus)

- **Profile:** The raspberry plant leaves are known for their medicinal properties.
- **Uses:** Widely used in herbal teas, especially for pregnant women, to strengthen and tone the uterus, potentially easing labour. Also used for menstrual cramps, gastrointestinal disorders, and as a general tonic for the reproductive system.

Red Clover (Trifolium pratense)

- **Profile:** A perennial herbaceous plant with small, pinkish-purple flowers.
- **Uses:** Used for menopausal symptoms like hot flashes and night sweats due to its phytoestrogen content. Also believed to improve cardiovascular health and bone density. Applied topically, it can help with skin inflammations and irritations.

Red Poppy (Papaver rhoeas)

- **Profile:** A flowering plant with bright red, delicate petals.
- **Uses:** The petals have mild sedative properties and are used in herbal preparations to ease coughs and promote sleep.

Red Sage (Salvia miltiorrhiza)

- **Profile:** Also known as Danshen, it's a perennial plant with purple flowers used in traditional Chinese medicine.
- **Uses:** Used to improve blood circulation, treat cardiovascular diseases, and for its anti-inflammatory effects.

Rehmannia (Rehmannia glutinosa)

- **Profile:** A perennial herb in Chinese medicine known for its large, purplish flowers.
- **Uses:** Used for its anti-inflammatory properties, to treat autoimmune diseases, and to balance hormones. Also known for supporting kidney health.

Rhatany (Krameria lappacea)

- **Profile:** A root traditionally used in herbal medicine.
- **Uses:** The root is used for its astringent properties, treating diarrhoea, and topical application for skin irritations and bleeding gums.

Rhodiola (Rhodiola rosea)

- **Profile:** A herb growing in cold, mountainous regions of Europe and Asia.
- **Uses:** Known as an adaptogen, it's used to reduce fatigue, enhance mental performance, and help the body adapt to stress. Also used for depression and anxiety.

Rock Samphire (Crithmum maritimum)

- **Profile:** A succulent, salty plant that grows on rocky shores.
- **Uses:** Traditionally used as a diuretic to relieve digestive issues.

Rooibos (Aspalathus linearis)

- **Profile:** A shrub native to South Africa, used to make an herbal tea.
- **Uses:** Rooibos tea is caffeine-free and rich in antioxidants. It's consumed for its potential to improve heart health, manage diabetes, and soothe digestive issues. Also used for its anti-inflammatory and antiviral properties.

Rosehip (Rosa canina)

- **Profile:** The fruit of the rose plant is rich in vitamin C.
- **Uses:** Consumed for its high vitamin C content and antioxidants. Used in herbal remedies to boost the immune system, improve skin health, and reduce inflammation. Also used for osteoarthritis and joint health.

Rosemary (Rosmarinus officinalis)

- **Profile:** A fragrant evergreen herb used in cooking and traditional medicine.
- **Uses:** Rosemary improves memory and concentration, promotes hair growth, and relieves muscle pain and spasms. It's also used for its antioxidant and anti-inflammatory properties.

Rue (Ruta graveolens)

- **Profile:** A garden herb with a strong, bitter taste and a potent scent.
- **Uses:** Traditionally used for its antispasmodic properties to treat conditions like cramps and muscle spasms. Also used for menstrual disorders and as a mild sedative. Due to its potency, it should be used with caution.

Rupturewort (Herniaria glabra)

- **Profile:** A low-growing plant traditionally used in herbal medicine.
- **Uses:** Used for urinary tract conditions such as kidney stones and bladder infections due to its diuretic properties.

HERBS S: PROFILES AND USES

Saffron (Crocus sativus)

- **Profile: A spice derived from the flowers of the saffron crocus, known for its distinctive golden colour and flavour.**
- **Uses: Used in cooking for its unique flavour and colour.** Medicinally, it's known for its mood-enhancing properties, often used to treat mild to moderate depression. Also used for its antioxidant and anti-inflammatory benefits.

Sage (Salvia officinalis)

- **Profile:** An aromatic herb with greyish leaves and blue-to-purplish flowers.
- **Uses:** Used in cooking and herbal teas. Medicinally, sage is known for its antioxidant properties and as a remedy for digestive problems, sore throats, and memory improvement.

Sanicle (Sanicula europaea)

- **Profile:** A woodland herb with clusters of small flowers.
- **Uses:** Historically used for its healing properties, particularly for wounds and respiratory conditions. It's also believed to have astringent properties.

Sarsaparilla (Smilax ornata)

- **Profile:** A tropical plant known for its root, which has a pleasant, slightly spicy flavor.
- **Uses:** Traditionally used to purify the blood, treat skin diseases, and as a diuretic. It's also used for its anti-inflammatory properties and in bodybuilding for its supposed testosterone-enhancing effects.

Sassafras (Sassafras albidum)

- **Profile:** A tree known for its distinct fragrance and three-lobed leaves.
- **Uses:** Traditionally used for its diuretic and stimulant properties. Sassafras tea was commonly consumed, though now it's regulated due to safrole content, a potential carcinogen.

Sassafras Bark

- **Profile:** The sassafras tree's bark contains a high concentration of safrole.
- **Uses:** Used in traditional medicine for treating skin ailments and rheumatism and as a flavouring agent in foods, though less common due to health concerns.

Saw Palmetto (Serenoa repens)

- **Profile:** A small palm native to the southeastern United States.
- **Uses:** Commonly used for benign prostatic hyperplasia (BPH) and to promote urinary tract function. Also believed to have anti-inflammatory properties.

Sea Buckthorn (Hippophae rhamnoides)

- **Profile:** A shrub producing bright orange berries, rich in nutrients.
- **Uses:** The berries, leaves, and seeds are used for their high content of vitamins and fatty acids. Known for promoting skin health, boosting immunity, and protecting against heart disease.

Sea Onion (Urginea maritima)

- **Profile:** A bulbous plant that grows near the sea.
- **Uses:** Used in traditional medicine for heart conditions due to its cardiac glycosides. It should be used with caution due to its potential toxicity.

Self Heal (Prunella vulgaris)

- **Profile:** A perennial herb known for its healing properties.
- **Uses:** Used to treat wounds and skin issues due to its antiseptic and anti-inflammatory properties. Also used for sore throats and mild internal inflammation.

Selenium

- **Profile:** A mineral essential for various bodily functions.
- **Uses:** Selenium is important for thyroid function and immune system health, and it acts as an antioxidant to protect against cell damage. It's also believed to reduce the risk of certain cancers.

Senega (Polygala senega)

- **Profile:** A plant native to North America, known for its roots.
- **Uses:** Used as an expectorant to treat chest congestion and respiratory infections. It has a stimulating effect on the mucous membranes.

Senega Snakeroot (Same as Senega)

- **Profile:** Also known as Senega, it's the root of the Polygala senega plant.
- **Uses:** Similar uses as Senega, primarily as an expectorant for respiratory conditions.

Senna (Senna alexandrina)

- **Profile:** A flowering plant used in traditional medicine.
- **Uses:** Mainly used as a natural laxative to treat constipation. It stimulates the muscles of the intestines to promote bowel movements.

Shepherd's Purse (Capsella bursa-pastors)

- **Profile:** A small plant with heart-shaped seed pods.
- **Uses:** Used to stop internal and external bleeding due to its astringent properties. Also used to treat urinary tract infections.

Siberian Ginseng (Eleutherococcus senticosus)

- **Profile:** A plant native to northeastern Asia, known for its woody root.
- **Uses:** Used as an adaptogen to help the body withstand stress. Also believed to boost energy levels, improve stamina, and enhance the immune system.

Silicon

- **Profile:** A naturally occurring element found in many plants.
- **Uses:** In dietary supplements, silicon is used to improve skin health, strengthen nails, and support bone formation.

Silverweed (Potentilla anserina)

- **Profile:** A perennial plant with silvery, feathered leaves and yellow flowers.
- **Uses:** Traditionally used for its astringent properties to treat diarrhoea and as an anti-inflammatory for joint pain.

Skullcap (Scutellaria lateriflora)

- **Profile:** A flowering plant known for its calming effects.
- **Uses:** Used to alleviate anxiety nervous tension, and to promote sleep. It's also used for its anti-inflammatory and antispasmodic properties.

Slippery Elm (Ulmus rubra)

- **Profile:** A tree native to North America, known for its mucilaginous inner bark.
- **Uses:** Used in herbal medicine to soothe the digestive tract, relieve sore throats, and as a mild laxative. Beneficial for inflammatory bowel diseases and acid reflux.

Soap Tree Bark (Quillaja saponaria)

- **Profile:** A tree native to South America, known for its high content of saponins in the bark.
- **Uses:** Traditionally used as a natural soap and shampoo. In herbal medicine, it's used for its expectorant and emollient properties.

Soapwort (Saponaria officinalis)

- **Profile:** A plant with clusters of pink or white flowers.
- **Uses:** The root is used for its natural saponins and has been used historically as a soap substitute for treating skin conditions.

Solomon's Seal (Polygonatum multiflorum)

- **Profile:** A plant with arching stems and tubular flowers.
- **Uses:** Traditionally used to treat respiratory conditions and as a general health tonic. Also used for joint and skin health.

Sorrel (Rumex acetosa)

- **Profile:** A leafy green plant with a sour, lemony flavour.
- **Uses:** The leaves are rich in vitamin C and used for their diuretic and appetite-stimulating properties. Traditionally used to treat scurvy and inflammatory conditions.

Soursop (Annona muricata)

- **Profile:** A fruit-bearing tree also known as Graviola.
- **Uses:** The fruit is eaten for its nutritional value. The leaves are used in traditional medicine to treat stomach ailments and fever and as a sedative. There is interest in its potential anticancer properties, though more research is needed.

Southernwood (Artemisia abrotanum)

- **Profile:** A shrubby herb with a strong aroma.
- **Uses:** Historically used as a vermifuge and to promote menstrual flow. Also used as an insect repellent.

Soy Isoflavones

- **Profile:** Compounds found in soybeans that have estrogen-like effects.
- **Uses:** Used to alleviate menopausal symptoms such as hot flashes and to promote bone health. Also believed to reduce the risk of heart disease and some cancers.

Spearmint (Mentha spicata)

- **Profile:** A species of mint known for its pleasantly sweet flavour.
- **Uses:** Used in cooking and herbal teas. Spearmint is known for its digestive benefits, as a remedy for nausea, and its mild sedative properties.

Spinach (Spinacia oleracea)

- **Profile:** A leafy green vegetable rich in vitamins and minerals.
- **Uses:** Consumed for its nutritional value, particularly its high levels of iron, calcium, and vitamins. Also known for its antioxidant properties.

Spikenard (Nardostachys jatamansi)

- **Profile:** A flowering plant of the Valerian family, known for its aromatic rhizome.
- **Uses:** Used as a soothing agent, similar to valerian. Also used traditionally to treat insomnia and anxiety.

Spirulina (Arthrospira platensis)

- **Profile:** A blue-green algae, often touted as a superfood.
- **Uses:** Used as a dietary supplement for its high protein content and rich array of nutrients. Believed to boost energy, support immune function, and improve cholesterol levels.

Scilla or Squill (Urginea maritima)

- **Profile:** A bulbous plant with medicinal properties.
- **Uses:** Traditionally used as a diuretic and expectorant. Used in small doses for respiratory conditions like bronchitis but can be toxic in large doses.

St. John's Wort (Hypericum perforatum)

- **Profile:** A plant with yellow flowers known for its medicinal properties.
- **Uses:** Widely used to treat mild to moderate depression. Also used for its anti-inflammatory properties and to promote wound healing.

Stevia (Stevia rebaudiana)

- **Profile:** A sweet-tasting plant used as a sugar substitute.
- **Uses:** Primarily used as a natural, low-calorie sweetener. Also believed to have antihypertensive and blood glucose-lowering effects.

Strawberries (Fragaria × ananassa)

- **Profile:** A widely loved red, juicy fruit.
- **Uses:** Consumed for their delicious flavour and nutritional value, particularly their high vitamin C content. They are also known for their antioxidant properties.

Star Anise (Illicium verum)

- **Profile:** A star-shaped fruit from an evergreen tree native to China.
- **Uses: Used as a spice in cooking for its liquorice-like flavour.** Medicinally, it's used for its digestive properties and relieves colic in babies.

Stinging Nettle (Urtica dioica)

- **Profile:** A plant known for its irritating hairs that cause a stinging sensation.
- **Uses:** Used for its anti-inflammatory properties, particularly for arthritis and allergies. Also used to support urinary health and as a nutritive tonic due to its high mineral content.

Strophanthus Seeds (Strophanthus spp.)

- **Profile:** Seeds from a genus of flowering plants, some species of which are used medicinally.
- **Uses:** Contains cardiac glycosides and has been used to treat heart conditions. Due to its potential toxicity, it's used under medical supervision.

Styrax (Styrax officinalis)

- **Profile:** A genus of shrubs and trees that produce a resin known as storax.
- **Uses:** The resin is used in perfumery and is traditionally used for its antiseptic and expectorant properties.

Sumac (Rhus coriaria)

- **Profile:** A shrub producing deep red berries ground into a spice.
- **Uses:** Used as a spice in Middle Eastern cuisine. Medicinally, sumac is known for its antioxidant properties and may help lower blood sugar levels.

Summery Savory (Satureja hortensis)

- **Profile:** An annual mint family herb used in cooking and herbal medicine.
- **Uses:** Used for its digestive benefits and to relieve cramps. Also used as an antiseptic and antioxidant.

Sundew (Drosera spp.)

- **Profile:** A carnivorous plant with sticky, glandular leaves.
- **Uses:** Used in traditional medicine for respiratory ailments like bronchitis and asthma due to its antispasmodic and expectorant properties.

Sunflower (Helianthus annuus)

- **Profile:** A large, bright flower known for its edible seeds.
- **Uses:** Sunflower seeds are rich in nutrients for their health-promoting fats, protein, and fibre. Sunflower oil is used for its skin health benefits.

Swamp Beggar's Tick (Bidens pilosa)

- **Profile:** A plant with small white or yellow flowers, known for its burr-like seeds.
- **Uses:** Used in traditional medicine for its anti-inflammatory properties and to treat infections.

Sweet Flag (Acorus calamus)

- **Profile:** A plant with sword-shaped leaves and a fragrant rhizome.
- **Uses:** Used for its digestive stimulating properties and to soothe the digestive tract. Also used for its soothing effects and to improve cognition.

Sweet Grass (Hierochloe odorata)

- **Profile:** A fragrant herb used in Native American ceremonial practices.
- **Uses:** Used for its calming aroma. Traditionally used to treat coughs and sore throats.

Sweet Gum (Liquidambar styraciflua)

- **Profile:** A tree known for its star-shaped leaves and spiked fruit.
- **Uses:** The tree's resin, or storax, is used for its antiseptic and anti-inflammatory properties. Traditionally used to treat skin problems and respiratory conditions.

Sweet Orange (Citrus sinensis)

- **Profile:** The fruit of the orange tree is known for its sweet flavour.
- **Uses:** The fruit is rich in vitamin C and antioxidants. Orange peel is used for its digestive-stimulating properties and as a mild sedative.

Sweet Potatoes (Ipomoea batatas)

- **Profile:** A starchy, sweet-tasting root vegetable.
- **Uses:** Consumed for their high vitamins A and C content, fibre, and antioxidants. Believed to support healthy vision, immune function, and blood sugar regulation.

HERBS T: PROFILES AND USES

Tamarack (Larix laricina)

- **Profile:** A species of larch tree native to North America.
- **Uses:** The bark is used in traditional medicine for its astringent and antiseptic properties, often in treating skin conditions.

Tangerines (Citrus reticulata)

- **Profile:** A citrus fruit similar to oranges but smaller and sweeter.
- **Uses:** Consumed for their refreshing taste and nutritional benefits. Rich in vitamin C and antioxidants, tangerines are good for immune support and skin health. The peel is used in traditional Chinese medicine for digestive issues.

Tarragon (Artemisia dracunculus)

- **Profile:** A perennial herb in the sunflower family, known for its aromatic leaves.
- **Uses:** Used in cooking for its distinct, slightly bittersweet flavour. Medicinally, it's used for its appetite-stimulating and digestive properties. Also used to help alleviate sleep and menstrual problems.

Tea Plant (Camellia sinensis)

- **Profile:** The plant from which green, black, oolong and white teas are harvested.
- **Uses:** Rich in antioxidants, tea is consumed for various health benefits, including enhancing mental alertness, aiding digestion, and potentially reducing the risk of heart disease and certain cancers.

Tea Tree Oil (Melaleuca alternifolia)

- **Profile:** An essential oil extracted from the tea tree leaves, native to Australia.
- **Uses:** Known for its powerful antiseptic properties. Widely used topically for treating acne, fungal infections, dandruff, and as a natural disinfectant. Also used in aromatherapy for its cleansing and rejuvenating effects.

Tribulus Terrestris

- **Profile:** A plant with spiky fruit used in traditional medicine.
- **Uses:** Commonly used to enhance sexual function and libido in both men and women. Also believed to improve athletic performance and body composition.

Thuja (Thuja occidentalis)

- **Profile:** Also known as arborvitae, an evergreen tree with a distinct fragrance.
- **Uses:** Used homeopathically for skin conditions, such as warts and polyps. Also used for respiratory tract infections.

Thyme (Thymus vulgaris)

- **Profile:** A Mediterranean herb with culinary and medicinal uses.
- **Uses:** Used in cooking for its strong, earthy flavour. Medicinally, thyme is known for its antimicrobial properties. It's used as an expectorant for respiratory conditions, to soothe sore throats, and in natural cleaning products.

Tongkat Ali (Eurycoma longifolia)

- **Profile:** A medicinal plant from Southeast Asia known as longjack.
- **Uses:** Used to increase testosterone levels, improve fertility, enhance physical performance, and reduce fatigue.

Toothache Plant (Acmella oleracea)

- **Profile:** An herb that numbs the mouth when the flowers or leaves are chewed.
- **Uses:** Used for dental pain relief and to reduce inflammation in the mouth.

Tormentil (Potentilla erecta)

- **Profile:** A herb with yellow flowers belonging to the rose family.
- **Uses:** The root is used for its astringent properties to treat diarrhoea and inflammation of the mouth and throat and to stop bleeding.

Tree Turmeric (Berberis aristata)

- **Profile:** A shrub with yellow wood and an important source of the compound berberine.
- **Uses:** Used to treat inflammation, eye infections, and digestive disorders. Berberine has been shown to have antimicrobial activity and to improve blood sugar control.

Tribulus Terrestris

- **Profile:** A leafy plant known for its spiky fruit.
- **Uses:** Often used to enhance sexual function and libido in both men and women. Also believed to improve athletic performance and body composition.

Trifid Bur Marigold (Bidens tripartita)

- **Profile:** A plant with yellow flowers and barbed seeds.
- **Uses:** Traditionally used for its anti-inflammatory properties and to treat colds and respiratory infections.

Turmeric (Curcuma longa)

- **Profile:** A bright yellow-orange spice commonly used in curries and mustards.
- **Uses:** Known for its anti-inflammatory and antioxidant properties. Widely used to alleviate pain, improve digestion, and as a natural treatment for skin conditions. The active compound curcumin is studied for its potential in preventing and treating various diseases.

Turkey Corn (Dicentra eximia)

- **Profile:** A flowering plant also known as a wild bleeding heart.
- **Uses:** It is not commonly used in modern herbal medicine but was historically used by Native Americans for various remedies.

HERBS U - Z: PROFILES AND USES

Uva Ursi (Arctostaphylos uva-ursi)

- **Profile:** Also known as bearberry, it's a small shrub with reddish berries.
- **Uses:** Used primarily for urinary tract health. It has antiseptic and astringent properties, effectively treating urinary tract infections, reducing inflammation, and promoting kidney health. It should be used under professional guidance due to potential side effects.

Valerian (Valeriana officinalis)

- **Profile:** A flowering plant with sweetly scented flowers and medicinal roots.
- **Uses:** Widely known for its soothing properties. Used to treat insomnia, anxiety, and stress-related symptoms. Also used as a muscle relaxant and in managing menstrual cramps.

Varuna (Crataeva nurvala)

- **Profile:** A tree used in Ayurvedic medicine, particularly the bark.
- **Uses:** Used to treat urinary tract disorders and kidney stones and to improve bladder and kidney function.

Vervain (Verbena officinalis)

- **Profile:** A perennial herb with small, pale lilac flowers.
- **Uses:** Used for its calming effect to relieve anxiety and stress and for digestive disorders. Also used as a galactagogue to increase milk supply in breastfeeding women.

Violet (Viola spp.)

- **Profile:** A genus of flowering plants with delicate, often purple flowers.
- **Uses:** Used for its mild laxative effects and to soothe the respiratory tract. Also used topically for skin conditions.

Virginia Snakeroot (Aristolochia serpentaria)

- **Profile:** A plant known for its use in traditional remedies.
- **Uses:** Historically used for respiratory and digestive disorders and as a stimulant. Contains aristolochic acid, which can be nephrotoxic and carcinogenic.

Wahoo Bark (Euonymus atropurpureus)

- **Profile:** A shrub native to North America, known for its dark red berries.
- **Uses:** The bark is used in small doses in traditional medicine as a laxative and a diuretic. Also used for liver and gallbladder issues. Due to its potential toxicity, it should be used cautiously and under professional guidance.

Walnuts (Juglans regia)

- **Profile:** A type of nut known for its rich nutritional profile.
- **Uses:** Consumed for their high omega-3 fatty acid content, which supports brain health. They are also known for their antioxidant and anti-

inflammatory properties, aiding heart health and diabetes management.

Wasabi (Eutrema japonicum)

- **Profile:** A Japanese plant known for its strong, spicy flavour, often used as a condiment.
- **Uses:** Besides culinary uses, wasabi has antimicrobial properties and may offer health benefits in terms of cancer prevention and cardiovascular health due to its high levels of glucosinolates.

Watercress (Nasturtium officinale)

- **Profile:** An aquatic plant known for its peppery flavour.
- **Uses:** Rich in nutrients, particularly vitamin K, watercress is consumed for its antioxidant properties. Used in salads and soups, it may benefit heart and bone health and has potential anticancer properties.

Wheatgrass (Triticum aestivum)

- **Profile:** The freshly sprouted leaves of the wheat plant.
- **Uses:** Consumed as a dietary supplement for its high nutrient content, including vitamins, minerals, and chlorophyll. Believed to detoxify the body, boost immunity, and improve digestion.

White Dead Nettle (Lamium album)

- **Profile:** A plant with white flowers resembling stinging nettles but without the sting.
- **Uses:** Used for its astringent and anti-inflammatory properties, particularly in treating menstrual complaints and as a diuretic.

White Horehound (Marrubium vulgare)

- **Profile:** An herb with woolly leaves and white flowers.
- **Uses:** Traditionally used as an expectorant to treat coughs and colds. Also used for digestive issues due to its bitter principles.

White Mulberry (Morus alba)

- **Profile:** A tree known for its fruit and leaves, the primary food source for silkworms.
- **Uses:** The leaves treat diabetes and regulate blood sugar levels. The fruit is rich in antioxidants.

White Oak (Quercus alba)

- **Profile:** A large tree native to North America, known for its strong and durable wood.
- **Uses:** The bark is used medicinally as an astringent, antiseptic, and anti-inflammatory agent. Traditionally used to treat skin irritations, haemorrhoids, and diarrhoea.

White Pepper (Piper nigrum)

- **Profile:** The ripe fruit seeds of the pepper plant, with the outer layer removed.
- **Uses:** Used similarly to black pepper, it aids digestion and has anti-inflammatory properties.

White Pine (Pinus strobus)

- **Profile:** A large pine tree native to North America.
- **Uses:** The inner bark is used for respiratory conditions, coughs, and colds due to its expectorant properties.

White Pond Lily (Nymphaea odorata)

- **Profile:** An aquatic plant with large, fragrant white flowers.
- **Uses:** The root is used in traditional medicine as an astringent to soothe gastrointestinal and genitourinary tracts.

White Willow Bark (Salix alba)

- **Profile:** The bark of the white willow tree is known for its pain-relieving properties.
- **Uses:** It contains salicin, a precursor to aspirin, and is used for its analgesic and anti-inflammatory effects, particularly for headaches and arthritis.

Wild Carrot (Daucus carota)

- **Profile:** Also known as Queen Anne's lace, the wild ancestor of the domestic carrot.
- **Uses:** The seeds are used as a diuretic to treat digestive issues. Also used historically for contraceptive purposes.

Wild Indigo (Baptisia tinctoria)

- **Profile:** A plant with yellow flowers and seed pods.
- **Uses:** Used as an immune stimulant and anti-inflammatory for its antiseptic properties, particularly for infections.

Wild Strawberry (Fragaria vesca)

- **Profile:** A plant with small, flavorful berries.
- **Uses:** The berries are high in vitamins and antioxidants. The leaves are used for their diuretic and astringent properties, often in teas for digestive health.

Wild Yam (Dioscorea villosa)

- **Profile:** A vine with tuberous roots used in herbal medicine.
- **Uses:** Traditionally used to relieve menstrual cramps and menopausal symptoms. Also believed to aid in digestion and help regulate blood sugar levels.

Willow Bark (Salix alba)

- **Profile:** Willow tree bark has historically been used for pain relief.
- **Uses:** Contains salicin, which is similar to aspirin. Used for its analgesic and anti-inflammatory properties to treat headaches, muscle pain, and arthritis.

Wintergreen (Gaultheria procumbens)

- **Profile:** A small plant with red berries known for its minty flavour.
- **Uses:** The oil is used for pain relief, particularly muscle and joint pain. It contains methyl salicylate, which is similar to aspirin.

Witch Hazel (Hamamelis virginiana)

- **Profile:** A shrub known for its astringent properties.
- **Uses:** Widely used topically for skin care, to treat irritations, and as a natural remedy for haemorrhoids.

Wood Avens (Geum urbanum)

- **Profile:** A perennial plant with yellow flowers and a clove-scented root.
- **Uses:** The root is used for its astringent properties to treat diarrhoea and aid digestion. It's also used for sore throats.

Wormseed (Chenopodium ambrosioides)

- **Profile:** Mexican tea is a plant with a strong, pungent odour.
- **Uses:** Historically used to treat intestinal worms and as a digestive aid. It contains ascaridole, which can be toxic and should be used with caution.

Wormwood (Artemisia absinthium)

- **Profile:** A herb with a bitter taste used to make absinthe.
- **Uses:** Known for its digestive stimulating properties. Used to treat digestive disorders and as a natural remedy for worm infestations. Due to its thujone content, it should be used with caution.

Yarrow (Achillea millefolium)

- **Profile:** A flowering plant with a long history of medicinal use.
- **Uses:** Used for its anti-inflammatory and astringent properties. Traditionally used to stop bleeding, heal wounds, and for its benefits in treating colds, fever, and digestive disorders.

Yellow Dock (Rumex crispus)

- **Profile:** A perennial herb with tall, curly leaves.
- **Uses:** Used as a digestive tonic to improve bowel function and its blood-purifying properties. Also used to treat skin conditions.

Yellow Loosestrife (Lysimachia vulgaris)

- **Profile:** A perennial plant with yellow flowers, not to be confused with purple loosestrife (Lythrum salicaria).
- **Uses:** Traditionally used for its astringent and anti-inflammatory properties and to treat wounds and gastrointestinal issues.

Yellow Parilla (Menispermum canadense)

- **Profile:** Also known as Canadian moonseed, it is a climbing vine with broad leaves.
- **Uses:** Native Americans used it traditionally for its diuretic and laxative properties and to stimulate digestion.

Yerba Mate (Ilex paraguariensis)

- **Profile:** A South American plant whose leaves are used to make a popular beverage.
- **Uses:** Consumed for its stimulating effect due to its caffeine content. It is believed to have antioxidant properties and is used to enhance mental focus, aid weight loss, and boost energy levels.

Yerba Santa (Eriodictyon californicum)

- **Profile:** A medicinal herb native to California.
- **Uses:** Traditionally used for respiratory health, including treating coughs, colds, asthma, and bronchitis. Known for its expectorant properties, helping to clear mucus from the lungs.

Ylang Ylang (Cananga odorata)

- **Profile:** A tropical tree known for its fragrant flowers.
- **Uses:** The essential oil is used in aromatherapy for its relaxing and mood-lifting properties. Topically, it's used for its potential to improve skin health, reduce inflammation, and promote hair growth.

CONCLUSION

As we conclude our extensive journey through the "Herbal Encyclopedia: The Complete A-Z Profiles and Uses of Medicinal and Culinary Herbs," we find ourselves enriched with a deeper appreciation and understanding of the natural world's treasures. This compendium has not just served as a guide to the diverse array of herbs and their uses but has also opened a gateway to integrating the wisdom of nature into our daily lives.

Throughout this encyclopedia, we've explored the multifaceted roles of herbs, from their traditional medicinal applications to their delightful culinary contributions. Each page has offered insights into herbs' history, benefits, and practical applications, revealing how these natural wonders can support health, enhance culinary creations, and enrich our overall well-being.

In our hands, we now hold a resource that transcends the mere identification of herbs. This book encourages a proactive approach to health and wellness, blending the age-old knowledge of herbal medicine with modern lifestyle needs. It equips readers with the tools to harness herbs' therapeutic and culinary potentials, promoting a lifestyle that values holistic health and natural harmony.

The "Herbal Encyclopedia" is a testament to the enduring relationship between humans and the plant kingdom. It highlights the need for continued learning, exploration, and respect for the natural world. As we integrate these herbal wonders into our health regimens and kitchens, we contribute to a legacy of wellness and natural living that benefits ourselves, the environment, and future generations.

Dear Cherished Reader,

As I sit down to write this note, I'm reflecting on the many evenings and early mornings spent in the quiet company of nature's wisdom, translating its silent language into the words that fill the pages of this book.

Alongside a team of editors and writers who share a reverence for the earth's healing touch—we've woven together a guide we hope will illuminate your path to wellness and harmony with the natural world.

Did this book help you in some way? I'd be honored to know.

Your story, your transformation, and the impact it has had on your life hold immeasurable value. A few words from you shared as a review would warm my heart and serve as a guiding star for others searching for the same solace and strength in nature that you've found.

SCAN ME

SOURCES

https://www.webmd.com/balance/ss/slideshow-home-remedies

https://www.healthline.com/health/home-remedies

https://www.ncbi.nlm.nih.gov/pmc/articles/PMC3358962/

https://www.herbal-supplement-resource.com/medicinal-herbs.html

https://www.herbwisdom.com/herblist.html

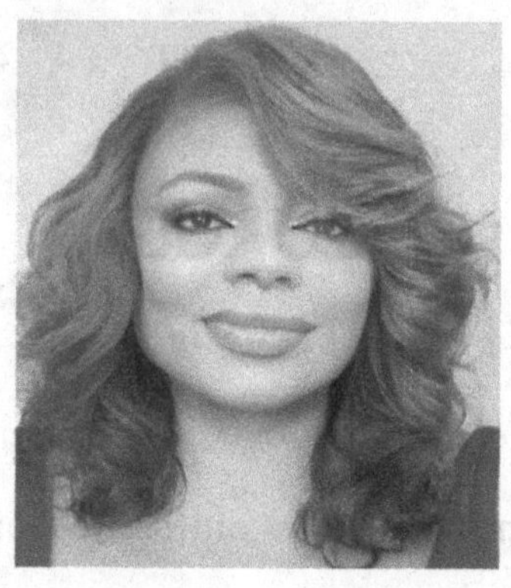

About the Author

Glorioustina Essia is a multifaceted professional whose expertise traverses the realms of technology, artificial intelligence, literature, and natural health. As a driving force in artificial intelligence, particularly in prompt engineering, she has established herself as a pioneer. Her proficiency extends to project management, network marketing, website development, and copywriting, showcasing a unique blend of technical understanding and creative flair.

A prolific author and publisher, Glorioustina's literary works span multiple genres, captivating a diverse audience with her narrative skill and inspiring a new generation of writers to unlock their creative potential. Her passion for storytelling matches her commitment to exploring and advocating for holistic health practices. Renowned in herbal medicine, she dedicates her life to studying and promoting natural health.

Glorioustina Essia's professional and personal journey is characterized by an unwavering dedication to her core strengths and a ceaseless pursuit of knowledge. Her zeal and expertise embody the limitless possibilities that arise from a commitment to innovation, quality, and a deep-seated passion for understanding the future of technology and the ancient wisdom of herbal medicine. Glorioustina is a testament to the power of interdisciplinary knowledge and its impact in a world where technology, literature, and natural health converge.

You can connect with me on:

🌐 https://www.amazon.com/author/glorioustina

Also by Glorioustina Essia

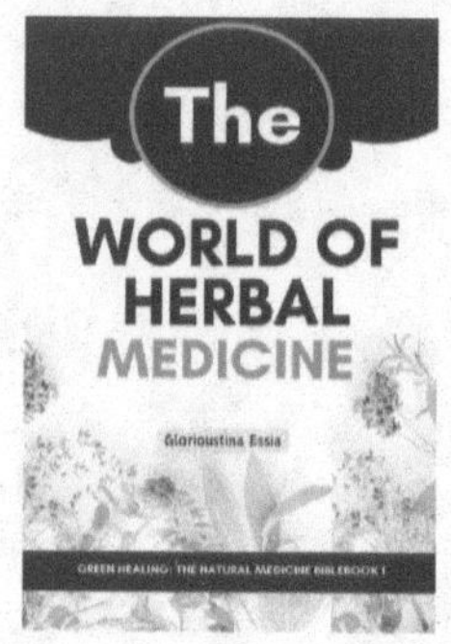

The World of Herbal Medicine

In an era where the rush of modern medicine often overshadows the pursuit of holistic health, the timeless wisdom of herbal remedies remains largely untapped. Do you find yourself seeking a more natural approach to health and wellness yet still determining where to begin or how to integrate these practices with modern healthcare?

Embark on a transformative journey with Book 1 of "Green Healing: The Natural Medicine Bible": "The World of Herbal Medicine." This enlightening volume takes you through the ancient pathways to the modern integration of herbal healing. Discover herbal medicine's rich history and evolution across different cultures, including the profound insights of Traditional Chinese Medicine, Ayurveda, and indigenous practices. Unravel how herbalism has evolved through historical epochs and how it beautifully intersects with modern medical practices today.

Embrace the journey to holistic health — add this captivating volume to your collection and begin exploring the world of herbal medicine today

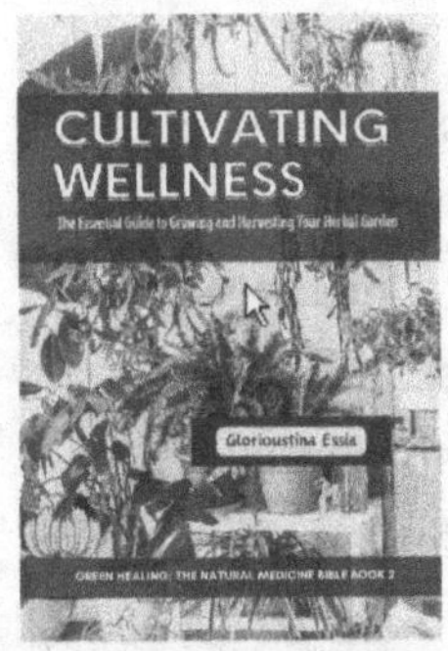

Cultivating Wellness

This guide is your gateway to mastering the art of herb gardening, offering practical advice for cultivating various medicinal and culinary herbs. From sustainable techniques to harvesting and preservation methods, each chapter brims with expert knowledge tailored to beginners and experienced gardeners. Learn to navigate common challenges in herb gardening and create specialized gardens for your health and culinary needs. Beyond gardening tips, this book inspires a deeper connection with nature and a commitment to a holistic lifestyle. Embrace the journey of nurturing not just a garden but a healthier, more harmonious way of life with "Cultivating Wellness."

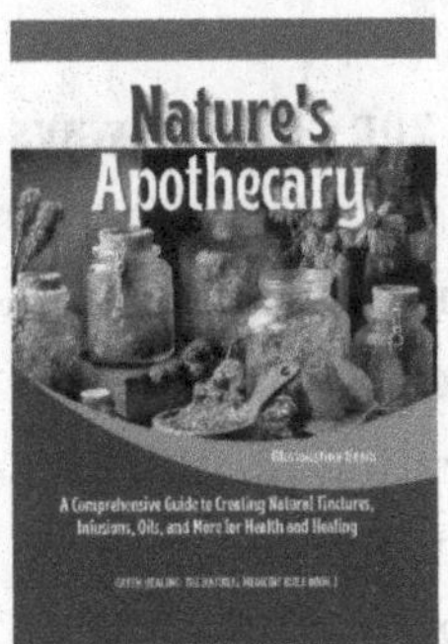

Nature's Apothecary

This comprehensive guide demystifies making your natural tinctures, infusions, oils, and more. It provides step-by-step instructions and detailed information on various herbs and their medicinal properties, empowering you to create effective, natural remedies in your kitchen.

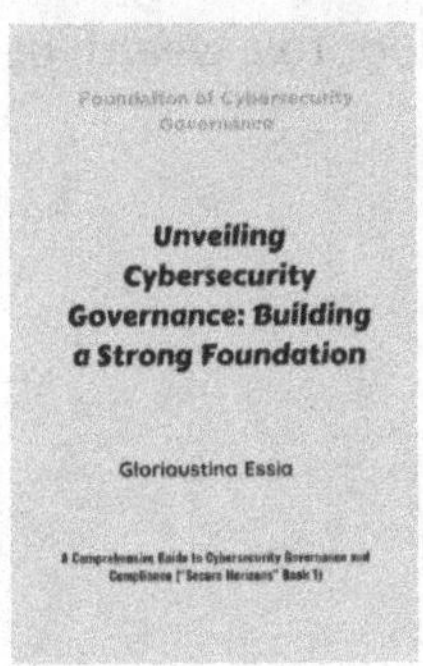

Unveiling Cybersecurity Governance

In the ever-expanding digital landscape, safeguarding sensitive information and maintaining robust cybersecurity practices have become paramount. "Unveiling Cybersecurity Governance: Building a Strong Foundation" is a comprehensive guide that delves into cybersecurity governance's core principles and components, equipping readers with the knowledge and tools to establish a secure digital environment.

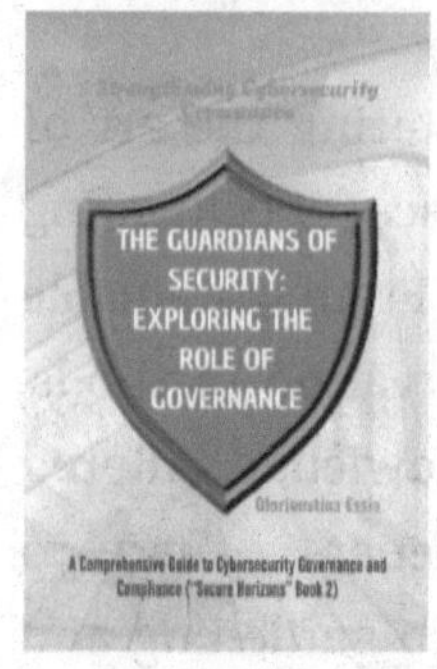

THE GUARDIANS OF SECURITY

Step into a world where cybersecurity governance catalyzes a secure future. Explore the realms of "The Guardians of Security: Exploring the Role of Governance," the much-awaited second book in the epic series "Secure Horizons: A Comprehensive Guide to Cybersecurity Governance and Compliance."

As you read each page of "The Guardians of Security," prepare to be enchanted by the author's remarkable storytelling ability. This book presents a vivid picture of the complicated landscape of cybersecurity governance with a seamless blend of real-world experiences, cutting-edge research, and visionary concepts. Immerse yourself in an exciting story that uncovers the brains and souls of people dedicated to defending our digital borders.

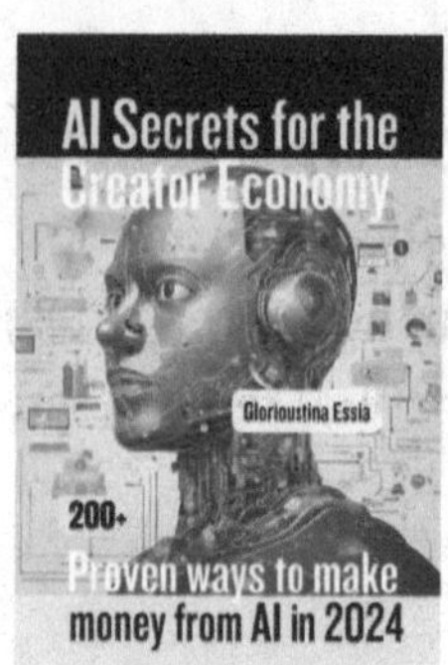

AI Secrets for the Creator Economy: 200+ Proven ways to make money from AI in 2024

In a world driven by innovation and transformation, the Creator Economy emerges as a powerful force, with Artificial Intelligence (AI) at its beating heart. This book, "AI Secrets for the Creator Economy: 200+ Proven Ways to Make Money from AI in 2024 and Beyond," is more than just a book; it's your key to unlocking the incredible synergy between AI and creativity, opening the door to a wealth of opportunities for those who are willing to seize them.